MANUAL OF COMMON BEDSIDE SURGICAL PROCEDURES

MANUAL OF COMMON BEDSIDE SURGICAL PROCEDURES

by the Halsted Residents of the Johns Hopkins Hospital

Editors

Herbert Chen, M.D.
Senior Resident in General Surgery
Fellow in Surgery
Johns Hopkins Hospital
Johns Hopkins University School of Medicine
Baltimore, Maryland

Juan E. Sola, M.D.
Chief Resident in General Surgery
Fellow in Surgery
Johns Hopkins Hospital
Johns Hopkins University School of Medicine
Baltimore, Maryland

Keith D. Lillemoe, M.D.
Associate Professor of Surgery
Johns Hopkins Hospital
Johns Hopkins University School of Medicine
Baltimore, Maryland

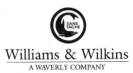

Williams & Wilkins
A WAVERLY COMPANY

BALTIMORE • PHILADELPHIA • LONDON • PARIS • BANGKOK
BUENOS AIRES • HONG KONG • MUNICH • SYDNEY • TOKYO • WROCLAW

Editor: Timothy S. Satterfield
Production Coordinator: Linda Carlson
Copy Editor: Bonnie Montgomery
Designer: Laura O'Leary
Illustration Planner: Ray Lowman
Typesetter: Peirce Graphic Services
Printer: McNaughton & Gunn
Binder: McNaughton & Gunn

351 West Camden Street
Baltimore, Maryland 21201-2436, USA
1-800-638-0672

Accurate indications, adverse reactions, and dosage schedules for drugs are provided in this book, but it is possible that they may change. The reader is urged to review the package information data of the manufacturers of the medications mentioned.

Printed in the United States of America

Library of Congress Cataloging in Publication Data

Manual of common bedside surgical procedures by the Halsted residents of the John Hopkins Hospital / editors, Herbert Chen, Juan E. Sola, Keith D. Lillemoe.
    p.   cm.
    Includes bibliographical references and index.
    ISBN 0-683-01549-4
    1. Surgery, Minor—Handbooks, manuals, etc.   2. Clinical medicine—Hand-
books, manuals, etc.   3. Johns Hopkins Hospital.   I. Chen, Herbert.   II. Sola,
Juan E.   III. Lillemoe, Keith D.
    [DNLM: 1. Surgery, Operative—methods.   WO 500 M294 1995]
    RD111.M36   1995
    617'.024—dc20
    DNLM/DLC
    for Library of Congress

The Publishers have made every effort to trace the copyright holders for borrowed material. If they have inadvertently overlooked any, they will be pleased to make the necessary arrangements at the first opportunity.

95 96 97 98 99
1 2 3 4 5 6 7 8 9 10

Reprints of chapters may be purchased from Williams & Wilkins in quantities of 100 or more. Call Isabella Wise in the Special Sales Department, (800) 358-3583.

For Harriet, Leda, and Cheryl

CONTENTS

FOREWORD

This manual should fill very nicely a niche where currently no publication exists. There are many procedures that the junior surgical house officer is required to master. Generally these skills are acquired by on-the-job training. This manual provides the background information, and the step by step detail of technique, that are required if a young house officer is to acquire these skills, without a risky and dangerous learning curve. There are many outstanding surgical publications that describe the presentation, pathogenesis, diagnosis, and management of surgical diseases. In addition, there are a variety of surgical handbooks that are small enough to be portable, that in outline fashion provide information that the young surgeon requires to participate in the care of surgical diseases. There are no publications, however, that completely or clearly outline the technical and procedural information for which the junior surgeon in training is specifically responsible. In most instances institutions require young surgeons to have these skills without a formal training program. This book will fill that void.

All surgeons who are fortunate enough to practice in a teaching hospital recognize the abilities and skills that young surgeons in training have as teachers. During my 25 years on the full-time faculty of the Department of Surgery at The Johns Hopkins Medical Institutions, I have learned far more from the surgical house staff than I have taught them. The personality traits that lead young men and women into the field of surgery are also characteristics that make them outstanding teachers. This manual reflects the teaching skills of our surgical house staff and is solely the product of their efforts. The concept of creating this manual and its driving force has been the two surgical residents who have served as editors, Dr. Herb Chen and Dr. Juan E. Sola, who, while overseen by Dr. Keith Lillemoe, our residency program coordinator, deserve credit for the planning, development, and completion of this fine work. This publication should be of great value not only to young surgical house staff, but also house staff in other disciplines.

John L. Cameron, M.D.
March 1995

PREFACE

As the care of patients continues to become more complex and technologically oriented, there has been an increase in the number of invasive monitoring, diagnostic, and therapeutic procedures performed at the bedside. In many situations, these procedures are performed by surgical house officers on an elective and sometimes emergent basis. Although surgical residents will acquire the skills to perform the procedures by experience and "hands-on" instruction, a manual detailing and carefully illustrating the many diverse procedures would be beneficial. Currently, techniques for performing some bedside procedures can be found in subspecialty texts, but there is no convenient manual solely devoted to bedside procedures including techniques from a variety of medical fields.

Manual of Common Bedside Surgical Procedures is a useful, transportable, and fully illustrated text that attempts to accomplish this goal. The chapters on airway management and arterial/venous access are crucial to all house officers. Cardiothoracic, abdominal, and needle biopsy procedure chapters are especially useful to surgical residents. The chapters covering neurosurgical, urologic, plastic surgical, and orthopedic procedures can serve as quick references for intermittently performed procedures. Junior residents and medical students will find this entire manual to be a useful tool while first learning these procedures.

Manual of Common Bedside Surgical Procedures is edited by two current and one former Halsted resident. The chapters are written by the house officers of the Johns Hopkins Hospital, including Halsted surgical residents. The technical aspects of and the systematic approach to performing bedside procedures have been passed down from one resident to another over the years. By having residents as authors, the individuals actually performing these techniques are imparting important, first-hand knowledge targeted to other residents who will be performing these tasks. It was the dedication of these residents that made this book possible.

This text in no way aims to replace the "hands-on" instruction and experience needed to be accumulated by an individual prior to performing bedside procedures. No one should attempt a technique if they do not have adequate experience or supervision. Finally, the techniques described in this manual reflect the experience of the chapter authors, and may need to be be modified depending on each individual resident and each patient.

H. C.
J. E. S.
K. D. L.

ACKNOWLEDGMENTS

Manual of Common Bedside Surgical Procedures represents the dedication and hard work of the contributors. We are thankful for their expertise and efforts in providing important "tips" in performing bedside procedures. While the authors have written detailed instructions on performing these techniques, this manual would not be complete without precise illustrations. We sincerely thank our illustrator, Kimberly Battista, for her enthusiasm, persistence, and artistic talent. She definitely accommodated the busy schedules of these residents.

Several individuals helped us along the way in the production, support, and review of this manual. We thank them for their assistance and advice. These people include: Catherine Marcucci, M.D., Douglas W. Ball, M.D., Robert Udelsman, M.D., Jeffrey Kirsch, M.D., Steve Docimo, M.D., James Michelson, M.D., H. Kim Lyerly, M.D., and Linda W. Tracy.

Williams & Wilkins has been very supportive of our efforts. We and the contributors would like to thank Nancy Evans, Tim Satterfield, and Pat Coryell.

John L. Cameron, M.D., the Chairman of the Department of Surgery and Surgeon-in-Chief of the Johns Hopkins Hospital, provided much encouragement and advice throughout the production of this manual. We especially thank him for this, as well as his dedication to teaching the surgical house staff.

Finally, our efforts would not be possible without the support of our families. We sincerely appreciate their understanding and devotion.

CONTRIBUTORS

All contributors are from the Johns Hopkins Hospital and the Johns Hopkins University School of Medicine, Baltimore, Maryland.

Stephen A. Barnes, M.D.
Chief Resident in General Surgery, Fellow in Surgery

Herbert Chen, M.D.
Senior Resident in General Surgery, Fellow in Surgery

Elizabeth A. Davis, M.D.
Senior Resident in General Surgery, Fellow in Surgery

Jay H. Epstein, M.D.
Resident in Anesthesia and Critical Care Medicine

Cora Lee Foster, M.D.
Nutrition Support Fellow, Department of Surgery

Peter J. Gruber, M.D., Ph.D.
Senior Resident in General Surgery, Fellow in Surgery

Paul P. Lin, M.D.
Assistant Chief of Service and Instructor, Department of Surgery

Jennifer M. Lindsey, M.D.
Senior Resident in Orthopedic Surgery

Catherine Marcucci, M.D.
Fellow in Anesthesia and Critical Care Medicine

Peter Mattei, M.D.
Chief Resident in General Surgery, Fellow in Surgery

Attila Nakeeb, M.D.
Senior Resident in General Surgery, Fellow in Surgery

Thomas J. Polascik, M.D.
Senior Resident in Urologic Surgery

Prakash Sampath, M.D.
Senior Resident in Neurological Surgery

C. Max Schmidt, M.D., M.B.A.
Senior Resident in General Surgery, Fellow in Surgery

Juan E. Sola, M.D.
Chief Resident in General Surgery, Fellow in Surgery

Bernadette H. Wang, M.D.
Senior Resident in General Surgery, Fellow in Surgery

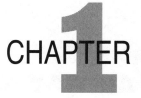

CHAPTER 1

AIRWAY MANAGEMENT

Authors: Catherine Marcucci, M.D. and Juan E. Sola, M.D.

AIRWAY MANAGEMENT

The establishment and management of a patent airway is the first principle of resuscitation and life support; it is an essential skill for all house officers. This skill is predicated on a thorough knowledge of airway anatomy.

A. MANUAL AIRWAY MANEUVERS—HEAD TILT AND JAW THRUST

1. Indications:
   a. Initial management of a compromised airway
   b. Stimulus to respiratory drive in the sedated patient
   c. Relief of mild anatomic airway obstruction (snoring, etc.)

2. Contraindications (to Head Tilt):
   a. Suspected cervical spine injury
   b. Down's syndrome (due to incomplete C1–C2 ossification and cervical vertebral subluxation)
   c. Previous cervical fusion
   d. Known cervical spine pathology (ankylosing spondylitis, arthritis, rheumatoid arthritis)

3. Anesthesia:
   None

4. Equipment:
   None

5. Positioning:

Supine

6. Technique—Head Tilt:

a. If any of the contraindications above apply, use jaw thrust only.
b. Tilt head back on atlanto-occipital (C1) joint while keeping mouth closed; head remains in neutral position.
c. Lift chin to facilitate elevation and anterior movement of hyoid bone away from pharyngeal wall (Fig. 1.1).

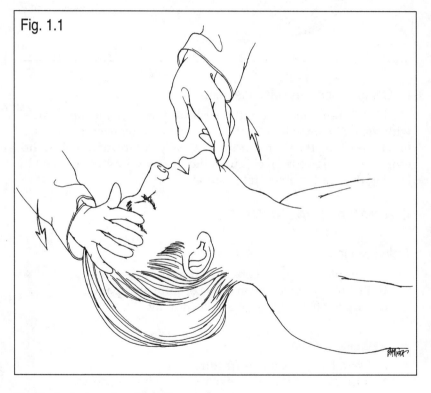

Fig. 1.1

7. Technique—Jaw Thrust:

a. Open mouth slightly, gently depress mentum with thumbs.
b. Grip mandibular rami with fingers and lift the mandibular teeth over and in front of maxillary teeth (Fig. 1.2).
c. A two-handed technique works best as the elasticity of the mandibular joint capsule and masseter muscle will pull the mandible back into the joint if the grip is relaxed.

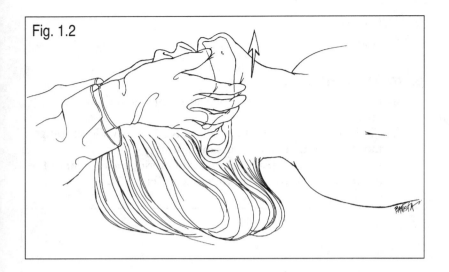

Fig. 1.2

8. Complications and Management:

In children under age 5, the cervical spine can bow upwards with manual maneuvers. Such maneuvers can worsen the obstruction by pushing the posterior pharyngeal wall upward against the tongue and epiglottis. In children, the airway is best maintained by leaving the head in a neutral position.

B. ORAL AIRWAY DEVICES

1. Indications:
    a. Complete or partial obstructed upper airway
    b. Bite block in the unconscious or intubated patient
    c. Adjunct for oropharyngeal suctioning

2. Contraindications:
    a. Dental or mandibular fracture
    b. History or acute episode of reactive airway disease

3. Anesthesia:
10% topical lidocaine spray to suppress gag response

4. Equipment:
    a. Plastic or elastomeric flanged oral airway

b. Tongue depressor
c. Suction apparatus

5. Positioning:

Supine or lateral

6. Technique:
   a. Open mouth; place tongue blade at base of tongue; draw the tongue anteriorly to lift it off the pharynx.
   b. Place airway in the mouth with the concave side facing the mentum so that the distal end is approximating but not touching the posterior wall of the oropharynx; flange and 1–2 cm of the shaft of the airway should protrude above the incisors.
   c. Perform the jaw thrust maneuver to lift the tongue off the pharyngeal wall.
   d. Tap the airway down the last 2 cm so that the curve lies beyond the base of the tongue.
   e. Alternatively, the airway may be inserted with concave side facing the palate. Insert in mouth until tip is past the uvula (no tongue blade required); rotate 180° to sweep under tongue from the side. This method of twisting the oral airway in the mouth is *not recommended* if patient has poor dentition or oral trauma, as the teeth may be further dislodged or bleeding increased.

7. Complications and Management:
   a. Exacerbation of reactive airway disease
      • Maintain airway with maneuver described in section A.
   b. Retching or vomiting
      • Turn the head to the side and suction.
   c. Increased airway obstruction if not properly placed
      • Remove the device and re-insert if needed.

C. NASAL AIRWAY DEVICES

1. Indications:
   a. Upper airway obstruction in awake or semicomatose patients
   b. Dental or oropharyngeal trauma

c. Inadequate airway patency after placement of oral airway device

2. Contraindications:

a. Nasal occlusion
b. Nasal fractures or basal skull fractures
c. Deviated septum
d. Coagulopathy
e. CSF rhinorrhea
f. Previous transsphenoidal hypophysectomy
g. Previous posterior pharyngeal flap for repair of craniofacial defects
h. Pregnancy (due to vascular engorgement of the nasal passages after the first trimester)

3. Anesthesia:

a. Gauge patency of nares by visual inspection (relative size, presence of bleeding or polyps) or by exhalation test.
   - Have the patient exhale through nose onto small hand-held mirror or shiny bevel of laryngoscope blade.
   - Relative size of condensation indicates which naris is more patent.
b. Mix a slurry (generally 10 mg phenylephrine in 10 mL of 2% lidocaine jelly) to provide topical anesthesia and vasoconstriction of the nasal airway.
c. Swab lidocaine jelly mixture just inside external edge of nares until local anesthesia occurs.
d. Gently place successive swabs deeper into naris until 3 swabs can comfortably be placed simultaneously to the level of the posterior nasal wall.
e. If three cotton swabs can be accommodated, a 7.5 mm airway will usually pass.
f. If swabs are not available, the lidocaine mix may be syringed directly into the nose.

4. Equipment:

a. Cotton swabs
b. Graduated sizes of nasal airways (generally 6.0 to 8.0 mm)
c. 2% lidocaine jelly
d. Phenylephrine
e. Suction apparatus

5. Positioning:

> Supine, lateral, or sitting

6. Technique:

   a. Pass the airway gently into the nose with the concave side facing the hard palate.
   b. The airway follows a path through the nose that is parallel to the palate and under the inferior turbinate.
   c. If resistance is met in the posterior pharynx, bend the tube 60–90° with gentle pressure to proceed down the pharynx; it also may be helpful to rotate the airway 90° counterclockwise and rotate it back to the original position as it makes the bend down the pharynx.
   d. If the airway will not pass with moderate pressure, a narrower one should be used.
   e. If the airway still does not advance, withdraw it 2 cm and pass a small suction catheter through it, then push the airway forward using the catheter as a guide.
   f. If still unsuccessful, the naris can be re-dilated or the other naris can be prepped and used.

7. Complications and Management:

   a. Epistaxis
      • Pack anterior superficial bleeders per Section H.
      • Consult ENT service for posterior bleeding.
   b. Submucosal tunneling
      • Remove device.
      • Patient may require plastic surgical repair.

D. BAG-MASK VENTILATION

1. Indications:

   a. Spontaneous ventilation absent or inadequate
   b. Preliminary preoxygenation when intubation is planned
   c. Short-term oxygenation when ventilation is temporarily compromised

2. Contraindications:

   a. Hiatal hernia
   b. Suspicion of active or passive regurgitation

   c. Need to avoid head and neck manipulation
   d. Tracheo-esophageal fistula
   e. Tracheal fracture or laceration
   f. Facial fractures or trauma
   g. Severe disruption of dermal surface
   h. Full stomach (relative)

3. Anesthesia:

None

4. Equipment:

   a. Fitted face mask with collar
   b. Respiratory or resuscitator (Ambu) bag
   c. O_2 supply
   d. Suction device

5. Positioning:

Supine, head in anatomic "sniffing" position

6. Technique:

   a. Place an oral (section B) or nasal (section C) airway.
   b. Hold the mask in the left hand; the thumb and index finger grip the mask around the collar with the body of the mask fitting into the left palm.
   c. Place the narrow end of the mask on the bridge of the nose, avoiding pressure on the eyes.
   d. Lower the body of the mask to the face so the chin section of the mask rests on the alveolar ridge.
   e. Seal the contact areas with the midsection of the face by pulling the mandible up into the mask with the curled fingers of the left hand and tilting the mask slightly to the right (Fig. 1.3).
   f. Deliver intermittent breaths with the right hand on the bag.
   g. In a spontaneously breathing patient, time the delivered breaths to coincide with the patient's inhalations.
   h. In the tachypneic patient, alternate the assisted breaths with spontaneous respirations.

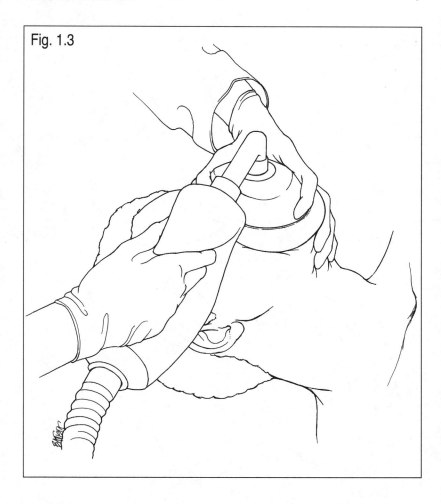

Fig. 1.3

i. Buccal gauze sponges can be placed in the cheeks of an edentulous patient to improve fit to the face. Care must be taken not to increase airway obstruction; if this occurs, remove sponges immediately.
j. In very difficult mask airways, the mask may be fitted to the face with both hands as an assistant delivers breaths (Fig. 1.4).

7. Complications and Management:
    a. Acute gastric distension requires placement of a nasogastric tube to decompress the stomach.
    b. Vomiting

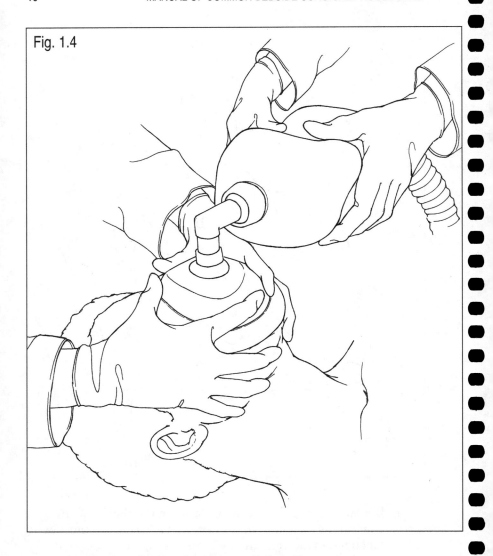

Fig. 1.4

E. TRACHEAL INTUBATION—ORAL AND NASAL

Nasal intubation is generally performed in the awake, spontaneously breathing patient when there is an advantage to avoiding laryngoscopy.

1. Indications:
   a. pO_2 decreased from age-appropriate level
   b. pCO_2 increased from baseline
   c. Change in mental status

d. In the adult patient, respiratory rate less than 7 breaths per minute or greater than 40 breaths per minute.
e. Inability to protect airway
f. Anticipated cardiovascular or respiratory collapse (sepsis, severe burn, etc.)
g. Anticipated bronchoscopic evaluation.

2. Contraindications:
   a. Oral intubation
      • Tracheal fracture or disruption
   b. Nasal intubation
      • Pregnancy (due to vascular engorgement of the nasal passages after the first trimester)
      • Coagulopathy
      • Nasal occlusion
      • Nasal fractures
      • Deviated septum
      • CSF rhinorrhea
      • Previous transsphenoidal hypophysectomy
      • Previous posterior pharyngeal flap for repair of craniofacial defects

3. Anesthesia:
   Frequently, an induction agent and a neuromuscular blocking agent are administered to facilitate intubation; a sedative is commonly given afterwards to lessen agitation in the awake, intubated patient.
   a. Induction agents
      • Thiopental (4–6 mg/kg)
      • Etomidate (0.3 mg/kg)
      • Ketamine (1–3 mg/kg)
   b. Neuromuscular blocking agents
      • Succinylcholine (1.0 mg/kg)
      • Vecuronium (0.3 mg/kg for rapid sequence induction)
   c. Sedatives
      • Diazepam (0.03–0.1 mg/kg)
      • Midazolam (0.05–0.15 mg/kg)
   d. Resuscitation drugs should be available at the bedside: atropine, phenylephrine, ephedrine, and epinephrine.
   e. Use topical lidocaine spray to anesthetize the airway when intubation of awake patient is planned.

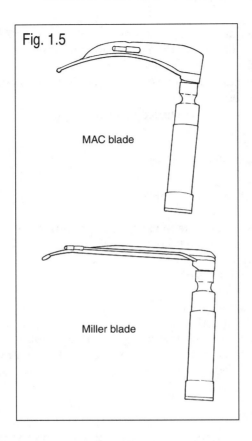

Fig. 1.5

MAC blade

Miller blade

4. Equipment:
a. Rigid laryngoscope blade and handle (Fig. 1.5)
b. Ambu bag and mask
c. O_2
d Suction apparatus
e. Styletted endotracheal tubes (ETT) in varying sizes (usually 6.0 to 8.0 mm for adults)

5. Positioning:
a. Supine with head in sniffing position if patient is already horizontal, unconscious, or if oral intubation is planned
b. May remain sitting for blind nasal intubation if the patient cannot tolerate lying flat

6. Technique—Oral Intubation:

   a. Check the ETT cuff for leaks by inflating and deflating the balloon with 10 mL of air.
   b. Check the blade and handle to insure the light is functioning.
   c. Pre-oxygenate with mask ventilation; have assistant apply cricoid pressure (Fig. 1.6).

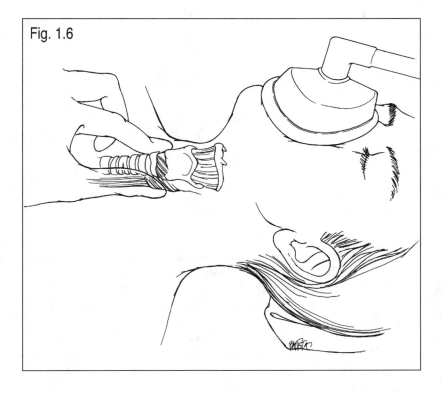

Fig. 1.6

   d. Remove oral airway.
   e. Grasp laryngoscope blade and handle in left hand.
   f. Instruct the awake patient to open the mouth as widely as possible. In the unconscious patient place the thumb and second fingers of the right hand on the right upper and lower molars and open the mouth with a scissor-like motion, subluxating the jaw out of the temporomandibular joint.
   g. Gently place the laryngoscope blade in the right side of the mouth, taking care to avoid damaging the teeth (Fig. 1.7).

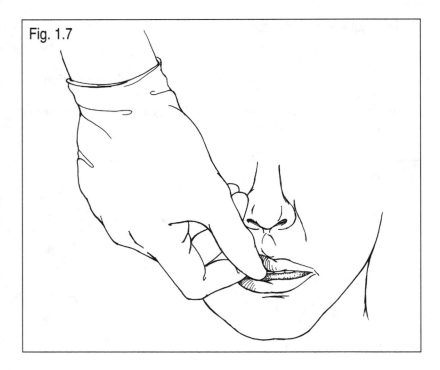

Fig. 1.7

h. Move the tongue to one side of the oral cavity while advancing the blade toward the glottic opening (Fig. 1.8).
i. Position the end of the blade under the epiglottis or in the vallecula, depending on the type of blade used (Figs. 1.9 and 1.10).
j. With the left wrist in an unbroken position, firmly lift the laryngoscope handle towards an imaginary point above the patient's left foot to expose the vocal cords. It is extremely important to *avoid* cocking the left wrist backward and levering the blade on the teeth.
k. Pass the styletted tube with the cuff deflated into the right side of the mouth and through the vocal cords; have an assistant remove the stylet as the cuff passes through the vocal cords to avoid damage to the trachea.
l. Place the endotracheal tube so that the cuff is just distal to the cords (cannot be seen between or above the cords); inflate the balloon with 5–10 mL of air and hold the tube firmly in place at the lips.
m. Place the portable end-tidal CO_2 monitor in the breathing cir-

Fig. 1.8

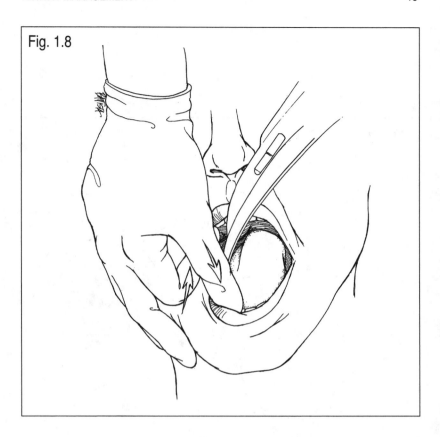

cuit between the tube adaptor and the ventilator bag; gently give several breaths. Watch the chest for expansion. Check a minimum of 6 breaths for measurement of CO_2 on the CO_2 monitor; this is to insure that CO_2 returned to the breathing circuit has a pulmonary source and is not insufflated air from the stomach. Listen for bilateral breath sounds over the chest and for an absence of sounds over the gastric area.

n. If all clinical signs point to intubation of the trachea, the assistant may release cricoid when instructed to do so.

o. *Tape the tube securely* and carefully place an oral airway or bite block in an awake patient to avoid obstruction of the tube by biting.

p. Obtain a chest X-ray to check ETT placement.

q. If more than one intubation attempt is necessary, the patient should have a mask airway re-established between attempts.

Fig. 1.9

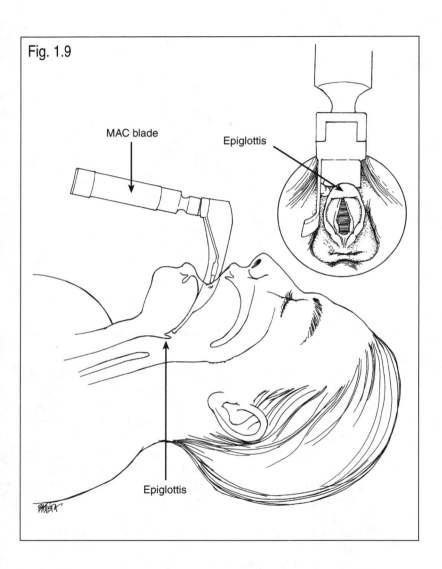

MAC blade

Epiglottis

Epiglottis

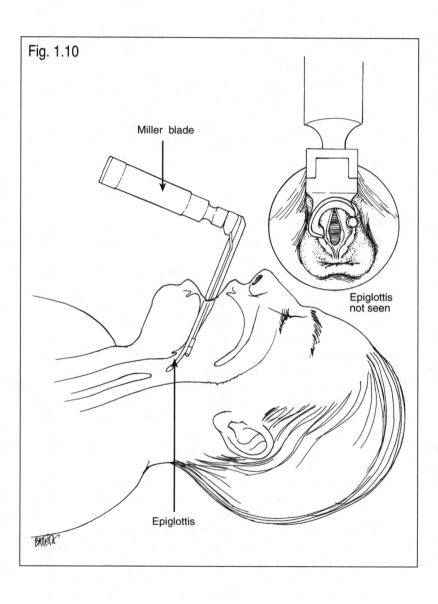

Fig. 1.10

Miller blade

Epiglottis
not seen

Epiglottis

r. If the esophagus is intubated inadvertently (in a case where the vocal cords are difficult to visualize), it may be helpful to leave the ETT in place as a "marker" to avoid repeated esophageal placements.

s. Inadequate mouth-opening is a common mistake and can make laryngoscopy unnecessarily difficult as well as greatly increase the risk of dental damage.

t. Exposure and visualization of the vocal cords is usually easier with a Miller blade but passing the ETT can be more difficult, as the view of the cords is sometimes obstructed by the tube as it passes through the oral cavity and supraglottis. Retraction of the right cheek and placing the ETT from the lateral side of the right molars can be helpful.

7. Technique—Nasal Intubation:

a. Check the ETT cuff for leaks by inflating and deflating the balloon with 10 mL of air.

b. Check the function of the laryngoscope light source.

c. Nasal intubation is generally done in the awake, spontaneously breathing patient when there is an advantage to avoiding laryngoscopy (cervical neck fracture, etc.)

d. Prep the nares as for a nasal airway.

e. Use nasal airways to dilate the naris; generally the endotracheal tube used will be one size smaller than the largest nasal airway that can be comfortably placed.

f. Coat the end and cuff of an unstyletted tube with viscous lidocaine jelly; if warm saline is available, the tube may first be soaked for 3 minutes and then preformed with a gentle curve about 3 cm from the end to facilitate passage under the epiglottis.

g. Place gently in the nose; advance the tube using the technique described for the nasal airway; gently extend the neck if the tube is difficult to pass.

h. Watch the tube for signs of "fogging" as the tube approaches the vocal cords; quality of the voice may also change (Fig. 1.11).

i. Ask the patient to breathe deeply and gently advance the tube through the cords while they are open during inspiration; the patient should immediately lose phonation.

j. Inflate the cuff, verify position, and secure as for an oral endotracheal tube. An oral airway is not necessary.

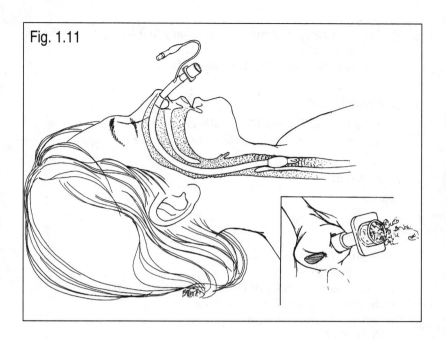

Fig. 1.11

8. Complications and Management:
    a. Minor airway damage
        • Inspect for lacerations to tongue, lips, and gums to ensure any bleeding has stopped.
        • Repair lacerations if necessary.
    b. Dental damage
        • Immediate retrieval of any dislodged teeth is mandatory.
        • Consult the dental or ENT service for further management.
    c. Esophageal intubation
        • Decompress the stomach.
    d. Major airway trauma
        • Obtain chest X-ray.
        • Perform emergent cricothyroidotomy if needed (Section F).
        • Consult the ENT service immediately.

F. SURGICAL CRICOTHYROIDOTOMY

1. Indications:

    Need to establish an emergent airway following:
    a. Extensive orofacial trauma preventing laryngoscopy

    b. Upper airway obstruction secondary to edema, hemorrhage, or foreign body

    c. Unsuccessful endotracheal intubation

2. Contraindications:

    a. Children under age 12. Needle cricothyroidotomy is preferred in order to avoid damage to cricoid cartilage.

3. Anesthesia:

None

4. Equipment:

    a. Scalpel blade and handle

    b. Tracheal spreader

    c. Tracheostomy tube or endotracheal tube (6–8 Fr.)

    d. Sterile prep solution, gloves, and towels

    e. Ambu bag and oxygen

    f. 3-O silk ties

    g. 2-O Prolene suture

    h. Hemostats

5. Positioning:

Supine with neck in neutral position. In trauma patients, care must be taken to protect the spinal cord as a *cervical spine injury must be presumed* until radiologic and clinical examination have excluded this diagnosis.

6. Technique:

    a. Sterile prep and drape the anterior neck if time permits (Fig. 1.12).

    b. Palpate the cricothyroid membrane below the thyroid cartilage in the midline.

    c. *Stabilize the thyroid cartilage firmly* with one hand and make a transverse incision approximately 2 cm in length down to and through the cricothyroid membrane. Inability to cannulate trachea can occur with creation of a false passage if cricothyroid membrane is not incised. This is best avoided by grasping the thyroid cartilage with one hand, thereby maintaining trachea in the midline, and carrying the incision down to and through cricothyroid membrane (Fig. 1.13).

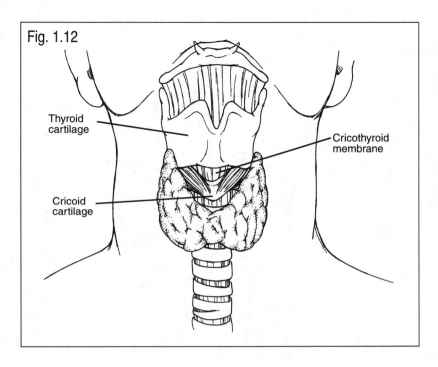

Fig. 1.12

Thyroid cartilage

Cricothyroid membrane

Cricoid cartilage

d. Insert tracheal spreader down the distal trachea and gently spread. Alternatively, if a *tracheal spreader is not available*, insert the handle of the scalpel transversely through the wound into the trachea. Rotate the scalpel 90° to enlarge the opening in the cricothyroid membrane.
e. With tracheal spreader in place, insert tracheostomy tube and remove tracheal spreader. Alternatively, a small retractor can be used if a tracheal spreader is not available.
f. Inflate cuff with 5 mL of air, attach Ambu bag, and ventilate patient with 100% oxygen.
g. Auscultate the chest to confirm equal and clear breath sounds bilaterally.
h. Control superficial bleeding either with direct pressure or with hemostats and 3-O silk ligatures if necessary.
i. Suture tracheostomy tube to skin with 2-O Prolene suture.

7. Complications and Management:
   a. Bleeding
      • Usually superficial and self-limited
      • Control with direct pressure or hemostats and ligatures.
   b. Esophageal injury

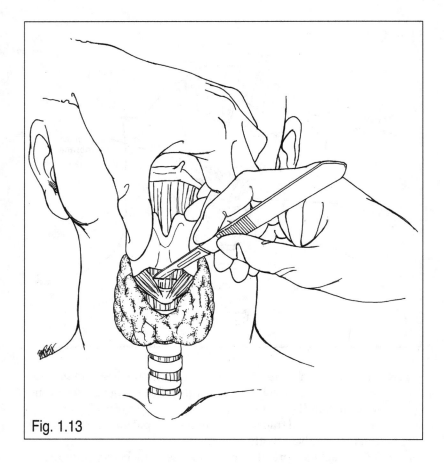

Fig. 1.13

- Can occur if scalpel penetrates the posterior trachea.
- Keep incision superficial, stopping once cricothyroid membrane is incised.
- If esophageal injury is suspected, obtain urgent surgical consultation.

G. NEEDLE CRICOTHYROIDOTOMY

Acceptable alternative to surgical cricothyroidotomy. However, needle cricothyroidotomy is a *temporizing measure* which can provide adequate ventilation for only 30–45 minutes.

1. Indications:

Need to establish an emergent airway following:
a. Extensive orofacial trauma preventing laryngoscopy

b. Upper airway obstruction secondary to edema, hemorrhage, or foreign body
c. Unsuccessful endotracheal intubation
d. Preferred method of obtaining emergent airway in children under age 12

2. Contraindications:

None

3. Anesthesia:

None

4. Equipment:

a. 12–14 gauge angio catheters
b. 3.0 mm pediatric endotracheal tube adaptor
c. Y connector
d. Oxygen supply with flow meter
e. Oxygen tubing
f. 5 mL syringe
g. Sterile prep solution and gloves

5. Positioning:

a. Supine with neck in neutral position. In trauma patients, care must be taken to protect the spinal cord as a *cervical spine injury must be presumed* until radiologic and clinical examination have excluded this diagnosis.

6. Technique:

a. Sterile prep and drape the anterior neck if time permits (Fig. 1.14).
b. Palpate the cricothyroid membrane below the thyroid cartilage in the midline.
c. Attach a 5 mL syringe to a 12–14 gauge angio catheter and puncture the skin in the midline over the cricothyroid membrane. Direct catheter *inferiorly at 45°* to the skin (Fig. 1.15).
d. Gently advance catheter while aspirating. Stop once air is aspirated, which confirms position within the tracheal lumen.
e. Advance the catheter over needle down the distal trachea and withdraw needle.
f. Attach 3.0 mm pediatric endotracheal tube adaptor to hub of catheter.

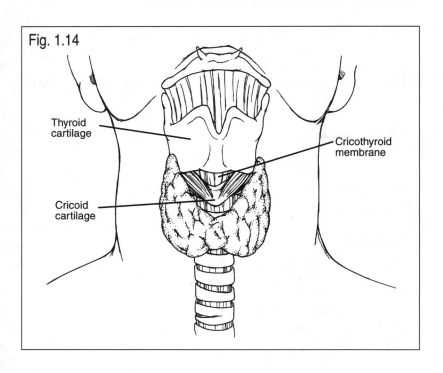

Fig. 1.14

Thyroid cartilage

Cricothyroid membrane

Cricoid cartilage

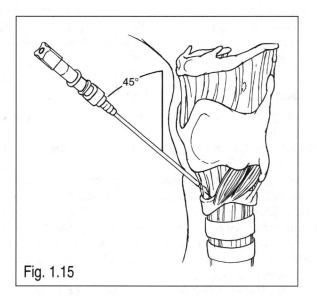

45°

Fig. 1.15

g. Attach Y connector to oxygen tubing and to pediatric endotracheal tube adaptor.

h. Maintain oxygen flow at 15 L/min.

i. Provide ventilation by intermittently placing thumb over
open end of Y connector for 1 second and off for 4 seconds.

7. Complications and Management:

a. Bleeding
- Usually superficial and self-limited
- Control with direct pressure or hemostats and ligatures.

b. Esophageal injury
- Can occur if angiocatheter penetrates the posterior
trachea.
- Stop advancing catheter once air is aspirated.
- If esophageal injury is suspected, obtain urgent surgical
consultation.

H. NASAL PACKS

1. Indications:

a. Persistent nasal bleeding despite simple first aid measures
and after clinical assessment has excluded shock.

2. Contraindications:

None

3. Anesthesia:

a. Cocaine solution (2.5–10%)

b. 1:1000 epinephrine

4. Equipment:

a. Headlight

b. Forceps

c. Suction catheter

d. Silver nitrate sticks

e. Lubricated ribbon gauze (0.5–1 inch)

f. Foley catheter

g. Syringe, 10 mL

5. Positioning:

Sitting

6. Technique:

a. Assess patient's general condition (BP and P) to determine effect of blood loss already sustained. Any patient who appears in shock should have a baseline hemoglobin, platelet count, PT, PTT, and cross matching of blood while resuscitation with crystalloid fluid is underway. In contrast, if the patient is hypertensive, reassurance and anti-hypertensives should be administered to control the blood pressure.

b. Stable patients should then be assessed sitting in a well-illuminated area where suction is available.

c. Initially have patient pinch nostrils between finger and thumb continuously for 10 minutes. Apply ice pack to bridge of nose.

d. If bleeding persists, remove blood clots from nose either with forceps or suction catheter.

e. Insert two cotton swabs soaked with 10% cocaine and 1:1000 epinephrine into bleeding nostril. This will anesthetize the nasal mucosa and vasoconstrict blood vessels.

f. Carefully inspect the nasal mucosa, searching for a bleeding point.

g. If bleeding has stopped, the patient should be observed for 1–2 hours to ensure that no further treatment is required.

h. If bleeding persists from a visible site, it should be chemically cauterized. After anesthetizing the area again with 10% cocaine solution, touch the bleeding point with a silver nitrate stick until hemostasis is achieved.

i. If bleeding continues without an identifiable source, nasal packing will be required.

j. Insert one end of the lubricated ribbon gauze (0.5–1 inch) along the floor of the nostril as far posteriorly as possible. Introduce sequential folds lengthwise from floor to roof of the nasal cavity until it is firmly filled. Generally, 100 cm of ribbon gauze can be inserted without difficulty (Fig. 1.16).

k. Pack may be left in place for 2–3 days with prophylactic oral antibiotics and ENT follow-up to remove pack.

l. If bleeding persists, a posterior nasal pack will be required. Remove anterior nasal pack and insert a Foley catheter along the floor of the nostril until the tip of the catheter reaches the nasopharynx (Fig. 1.17).

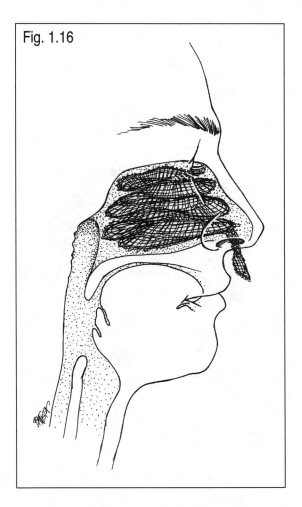

Fig. 1.16

m. Inflate balloon with 10 mL of air and withdraw catheter until balloon blocks posterior choana.

n. Tape catheter firmly to nostril to prevent balloon from falling into oropharynx.

o. Patient with posterior nasal packs will require hospitalization and prophylactic antibiotics.

7. Complications and Management

a. Persistent or recurrent bleeding
  • If anterior and posterior packs fail, surgical ligation of the maxillary and anterior ethmoidal arteries will be required.
  • Obtain surgical consultation.

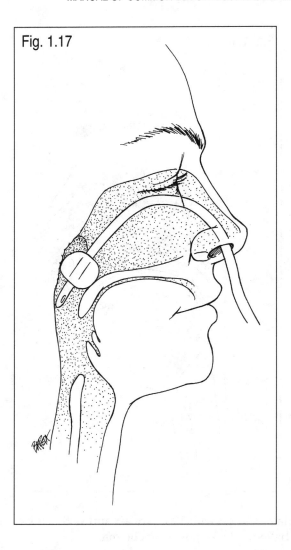

Fig. 1.17

b. Infection
  • Can occur with obstruction of the Eustachian tube.
  • Prophylactic antibiotics should be administered to pa-
    tients with nasal packs and instructions to seek medical
    care immediately for fever or discharge.
  • If infection is suspected, remove pack immediately.
c. Hypoxemia
  • May occur as nasal packs compromise respiration.
  • Elderly patients or those with respiratory problems should
    be admitted for observation.

CHAPTER 2

ARTERIAL AND VENOUS ACCESS

Authors: Herbert Chen, M.D. and Cora Lee Foster, M.D.

I. Central Venous Access
   A. Subclavian Venous Access
   B. Internal Jugular Access—Two Approaches
      1. Central Approach
      2. Posterior Approach
   C. Femoral Venous Access

II. Other Venous Access Procedures
   A. Peripherally Inserted Central Catheter (PICC), Long Arm IV
   B. Hickman Removal
   C. Greater Saphenous Venous Cutdown
   D. Intraosseous Access

III. Arterial Cannulation
   A. Radial Artery Cannulation
   B. Dorsalis Pedis Artery Cannulation
   C. Femoral Artery Cannulation
   D. Axillary Artery Cannulation

ARTERIAL AND VENOUS ACCESS

I. CENTRAL VENOUS ACCESS

Central venous catheters are frequently used in the ICU and operating room for monitoring and for venous access. Although this procedure is routine for most surgical houseofficers, central line insertion should be approached with caution and adequate preparation. Patient positioning is crucial to success.

A. SUBCLAVIAN VENOUS ACCESS

1. Indications:
    a. CVP monitoring
    b. TPN
    c. Long-term infusion of drugs
    d. Inotropic agents
    e. Hemodialysis
    f. Poor peripheral access

2. Contraindications:
    a. Vein thrombosis
    b. Coagulopathy (PT or PTT >1.3 ratio, platelets <20K)
    c. Untreated sepsis

3. Anesthesia:

1% lidocaine

4. Equipment:

a. Sterile prep solution
b. Sterile gloves and towels
c. 22 and 25 gauge needles
d. 5 mL syringes (2)
e. Shoulder roll towels
f. Appropriate catheters and dilator
g. IV tubing and flush
h. 18 gauge insertion needle (5–8 cm long)
i. .035 "J" wire
j. Sterile dressings
k. Scalpel
l. 2–0 silk suture

5. Positioning:

Supine in Trendelenburg. Place a towel roll between the scapulas underneath the thoracic vertebrae as shown. Allow the patent's shoulders to fall back posterior and caudal (or have an assistant apply gentle traction to the ipsilateral arm) (Fig. 2.1).

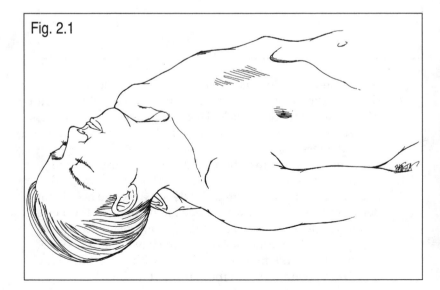

Fig. 2.1

6. Technique:

a. Sterile prep and drape the left or right subclavian area.
b. Place an index finger at the sternal notch and the thumb at the intersection of the clavicle and first rib (Fig. 2.2).

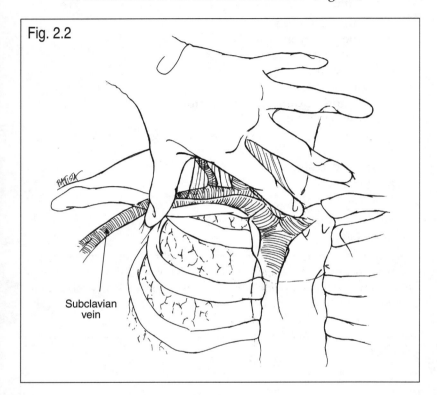

Fig. 2.2

Subclavian vein

Administer 1% lidocaine with a 25 gauge needle into the skin and subcutaneous area 2 cm lateral to your thumb, and 0.5 cm caudal to the clavicle. Use a 22 gauge needle to anesthetize the periosteum of the clavicle 2–3 cm lateral to the first rib intersection. *Always aspirate before injecting.*

c. Using the 18 gauge insertion needle with a 5 mL syringe, puncture the skin lateral to your thumb and 0.5 cm caudal to clavicle. While aspirating, slowly advance the needle underneath the clavicle toward your index finger at the sternal notch. *The needle must be horizontal (parallel to the floor) at all times* to avoid pneumothorax, and the bevel should be facing up. The needle may be depressed with your thumb if needed to get underneath the clavicle (Fig. 2.3).

d. *If no venous blood return* after advancing 5 cm, slowly with-

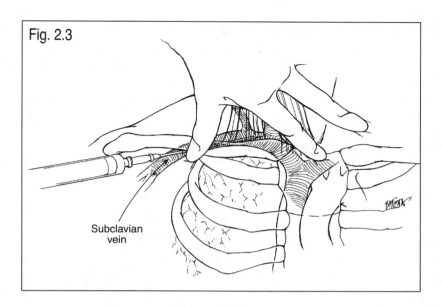

Fig. 2.3

Subclavian
vein

draw needle while aspirating (the needle might have punctured both vessel walls). If no blood return after completely
withdrawing needle, redirect needle aiming 1 cm above
sternal notch. If still no venous blood return, reanesthetize
the skin *1 cm more lateral* than previous site and attempt access at that site in the same manner as in (c). If still unsuccessful, stop procedure and consider trying the opposite
side after obtaining a portable chest X-ray to rule out pneumothorax.

e. *If air or arterial blood encountered,* stop immediately and see
   Section I.A.7 below.
f. If venous access obtained with good flow, remove syringe
   while keeping a finger over the needle to prevent air embolism.
g. Introduce the "J" wire, with the tip aimed towards the heart,
   through the needle while maintaining the needle in the
   same location (Seldinger technique). The wire must pass
   with minimal resistance.
h. If resistance is met, remove the wire, check needle placement by withdrawing blood with a syringe, and, if good
   flow is obtained, introduce the wire again while turning the
   patient's head to the ipsilateral side.
i. Once the wire is passed, remove the needle while keeping
   control of the wire *at all times.*
j. Enlarge the puncture site with a sterile scalpel.

k. Introduce the dilator over the wire 3–4 cm to *dilate the subcutaneous tissues only while keeping control of the wire.* Advancing the dilator the entire length can lacerate the subclavian vein and is *not* recommended (Fig. 2.4).

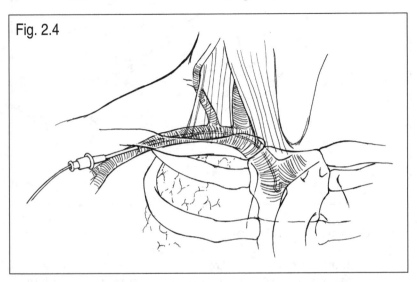

Fig. 2.4

l. Remove the dilator and introduce the central venous catheter over the wire to the length of *15 cm on the right and 18 cm on the left* (Fig. 2.5).

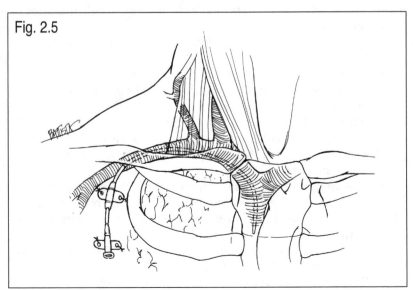

Fig. 2.5

m. Remove the wire, aspirate blood from all ports to confirm venous placement and then flush with sterile saline. Suture the catheter to the skin with silk suture. Dress the skin with a sterile dressing.

n. Run IV fluids at 20 mL/hr and order a portable chest X-ray to confirm placement into superior vena cava (SVC) and to rule out pneumothorax.

7. Complications and Management:

a. Arterial puncture
   - Withdraw needle immediately and apply manual pressure for 5 min.
   - Monitor hemodynamics and breath sounds for hemothorax.

b. Air embolus
   - Attempt to withdraw air by aspirating through catheter.
   - If hemodynamically unstable (cardiac arrest), initiate ACLS and stat thoracic surgery consult.
   - If stable, position patient in left lateral decubitus and Trendelenburg position to trap air in right ventricle. Chest X-ray in this position can demonstrate significant air and be used for follow-up.
   - Air will eventually dissolve.

c. Pneumothorax
   - If a tension pneumothorax is suspected, decompress with 16 gauge IV into second intercostal midclavicular space.
   - If <10%, 100% oxygen and serial 4-hour chest X-ray.
   - If >10%, tube thoracostomy.

d. Malpositioning:
   - Into right atrium (RA) or right ventricle (RV), against wall of vein—withdraw or advance as needed to place into SVC.
   - Into other subclavian vein—stable position, no adjustment needed.
   - Into jugular or mammary vein—re-introduce "J" wire, remove catheter, thread long 18 gauge IV catheter and confirm placement into vein by aspiration of blood. The "J" wire can now be redirected into SVC by maximizing positioning (pull caudally on arm and turning the head and neck ipsilaterally to close internal jug vein angle).

e. Dysrhythmias
   - Atrial or ventricular dysrhythmias are associated with

wires and catheters in the RA or RV and usually resolve
after withdrawing the catheter into the SVC.
- Persistent dysrhythmias may need medical management.

B. INTERNAL JUGULAR VENOUS ACCESS—TWO APPROACHES

1. Indications:

a. CVP monitoring
b. TPN
c. Long-term infusion of drugs
d. Inotropic agents
e. Hemodialysis
f. Poor peripheral access

2. Contraindications:

a. Previous ipsilateral neck surgery
b. Untreated sepsis
c. Venous thrombosis

3. Anesthesia:

1% lidocaine

4. Equipment:

a. Sterile prep solution
b. Sterile gloves and towels
c. 22 and 25 gauge needles
d. 5 mL syringes (2)
e. Appropriate catheters and dilator
f. IV tubing and flush
g. 18 gauge insertion needle (5–8 cm long)
h. .035 "J" wire
i. Sterile dressings
j. Scalpel
k. 2–0 silk suture

5. Positioning:

Supine in Trendelenburg. Turn the patient's head 45° contralat-
erally to expose the neck (Fig. 2.6).

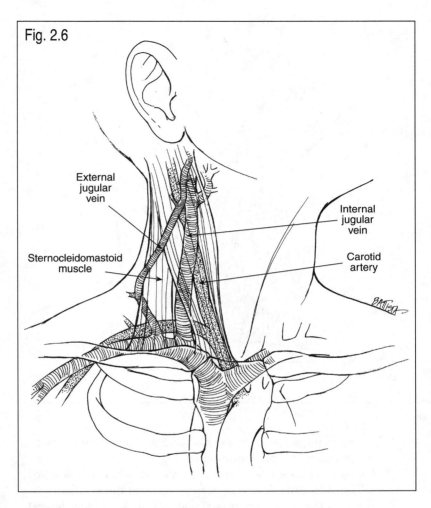

Fig. 2.6

External jugular vein

Internal jugular vein

Sternocleidomastoid muscle

Carotid artery

6. Technique—Central Approach:
   a. Identify the apex of the *triangle* formed by the heads of the sternocleidomastoid muscles (SCM). Also locate the external jugular vein and the carotid artery (Fig. 2.7).
   b. Sterile prep and drape neck.
   c. Administer anesthetic with 25 gauge needle into skin and subcutaneous area at the apex of the triangle. Always withdraw needle before injecting because the vein can be very superficial.
   d. Palpate the carotid pulse and apply gentle traction medially with the other hand.
   e. Insert the 22 gauge finder needle with a syringe at the apex

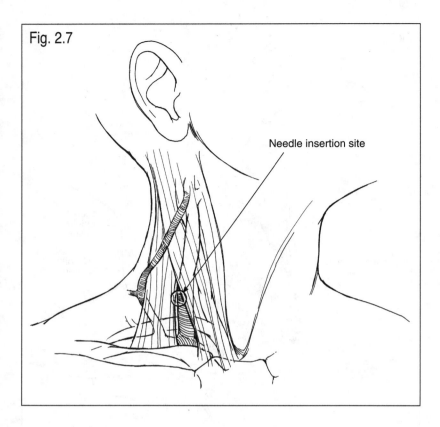

Fig. 2.7

Needle insertion site

of the triangle 45–60° to the skin and advance slowly toward
the *ipsilateral* nipple while aspirating.

f. *If no venous blood return after 3 cm,* slowly withdraw needle
   while aspirating. If still no return, redirect the needle
   through the same puncture site aiming 1–3 cm more lateral
   and then, if unsuccessful, 1 cm medial. *Watch the carotid
   artery.* If still no blood return, reassess landmarks and consider posterior approach if unable to obtain access after
   three attempts.

g. *If air or arterial blood encountered,* stop immediately and see
   Section I.B.8 below.

h. If good venous return, memorize the site and angle of entry
   of the finder needle and then remove the needle. Apply digital pressure to minimize bleeding. Alternatively, the needle
   may be left in place as a guide.

i. Insert the 18 gauge needle in the same manner as in (e) and
   (f) following the same angle as the finder needle (Fig. 2.8).

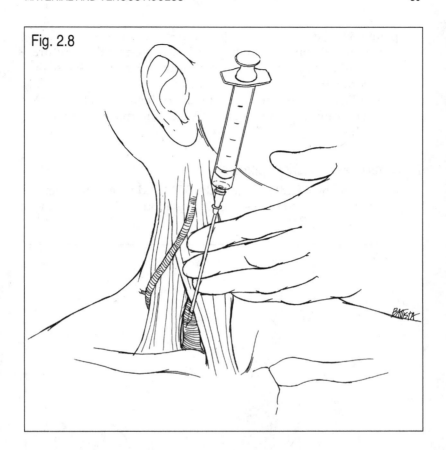

Fig. 2.8

j. If venous access obtained with good flow, remove syringe while keeping a finger over the needle to prevent air embolism.

k. Introduce the "J" wire, with the tip aimed towards the heart (medial), through the needle while maintaining the needle in the same location (Seldinger technique). The wire must pass with minimal resistance.

l. If resistance is met, remove the wire, check needle placement by withdrawing blood with a syringe, and reintroduce wire if good blood return.

m. Once the wire is passed, remove the needle while keeping control of the wire *at all times*.

n. Enlarge the puncture site with a sterile scalpel.

o. Introduce the central venous catheter over the wire while maintaining a constant hold on the wire to the length of about *9 cm on the right and 12 cm on the left.*

p. Remove the wire, aspirate blood from all ports to confirm venous placement, and then flush with sterile saline. Suture the catheter to the skin with silk suture. Dress the skin with a sterile dressing.

q. Run IV fluids only at 20 mL/hr and order a portable chest X-ray to confirm placement into SVC and to rule out pneumothorax.

7. Technique—Posterior Approach:

a. Identify the lateral border of the SCM and where the external jugular vein crosses over it. It is about 4–5 cm above the clavicle (Fig. 2.9).

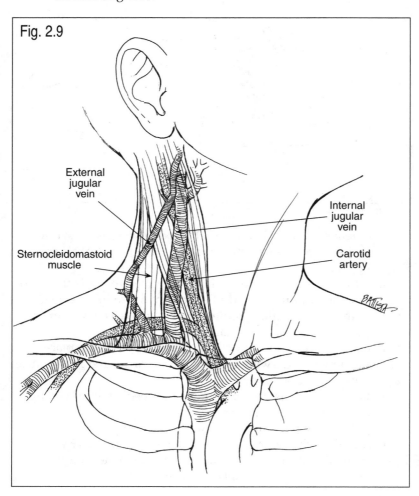

Fig. 2.9

External jugular vein

Sternocleidomastoid muscle

Internal jugular vein

Carotid artery

b. Sterile prep and drape neck.
c. Administer anesthetic with 25 gauge needle into skin and subcutaneous area 0.5 cm superior to the intersection of the SCM and external jugular vein. Always withdraw needle before injecting because the vein can be very superficial.
d. Insert the 22 gauge finder needle with a syringe at Point A and advance slowly *anteriorly and inferiorly* toward the sternal notch while aspirating (Fig. 2.10).

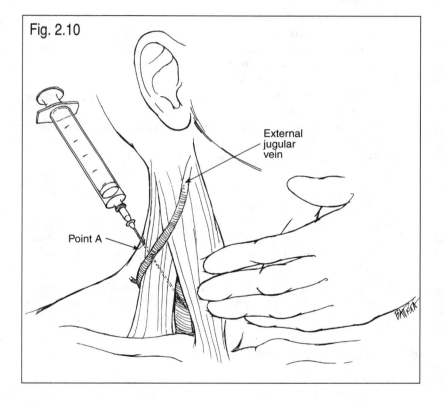

Fig. 2.10

External jugular vein

Point A

e. *If no venous blood return after 3 cm,* slowly withdraw needle while aspirating. If still no return, redirect the needle through the same puncture site aiming slightly ipsilateral to the sternal notch. If still no blood return, reassess landmarks and consider attempting the contralateral side if unable to obtain access after three attempts. *Chest X-ray must be obtained to rule out pneumothorax* before changing sides.
f. *If air or arterial blood encountered,* stop immediately and see Section I.B.8 below.

g. If good venous return, memorize the site and angle of entry of the finder needle and then remove the needle. Apply digital pressure to minimize bleeding. Alternatively, the needle may be left in place as a guide.

h. Insert the 18 gauge needle in the same manner as in (d) and (e) following the same angle as the finder needle.

i. If venous access obtained with good flow, remove syringe while keeping a finger over the needle to prevent air embolism.

j. Introduce the "J" wire, with the tip aimed towards the heart (medial), through the needle while maintaining the needle in the same location (Seldinger technique). The wire must pass with minimal resistance.

k. If resistance is met, remove the wire, check needle placement by withdrawing blood with a syringe, and reintroduce wire if good blood return.

l. Once the wire is passed, remove the needle while keeping control of the wire *at all times*.

m. Enlarge the puncture site with a sterile scalpel.

n. Introduce the central venous catheter over the wire while maintaining a constant hold on the wire to the length of about *9 cm on the right and 12 cm on the left*.

o. Remove the wire, aspirate blood from all ports to confirm venous placement, and then flush with sterile saline. Suture the catheter to the skin with silk suture. Dress the skin with a sterile dressing.

p. Run IV fluids only at 20 mL/hr and order a portable chest X-ray to confirm placement into SVC and to rule out pneumothorax.

8. Complications and Management:

a. Carotid puncture
  • Withdraw needle immediately and apply manual pressure.
  • If cannulation occurred and if manual pressure is not successful, then surgical intervention may be needed.

b. Air embolus
  • Attempt to withdraw air by aspirating through catheter.
  • If hemodynamically unstable (arrest), initiate ACLS and consider thoracotomy.
  • If stable, position patient in left lateral decubitus and Trendelenburg position to trap air in right ventricle. Chest

X-ray in this position can demonstrate significant air and be used for follow-up.
- Air will eventually dissolve.

c. Pneumothorax
- If tension pneumothorax, decompress with 16 gauge IV into 2nd intercostal midclavicular space.
- If <10%, 100% oxygen and serial 4-hour chest X-ray
- If >10%, tube thoracostomy

d. Malpositioning:
- Into RA or RV, against wall of vein—withdraw or advance as needed to place into SVC
- Into subclavian vein—stable position, no adjustment needed
- Into jugular or mammary vein—re-introduce "J" wire, remove catheter, thread long 18 gauge IV catheter and confirm placement into vein by aspiration of blood. The "J" wire can now be redirected into SVC by maximizing positioning (pull caudally on arm and turning the head and neck ipsilaterally to close internal jug vein angle).

e. Horner's syndrome
- Puncture of the carotid sheath can result in a temporary Horner's syndrome that usually spontaneously resolves.

e. Dysrhythmias
- Atrial or ventricular dysrhythmias are associated with wires and catheters in the RA or RV and usually resolve after withdrawing the object into the SVC.
- Persistent dysrhythmias may need medical management.

C. FEMORAL VENOUS ACCESS

1. Indications:
   a. Emergent central access
   b. Hemodialysis
   c. Unable to obtain subclavian or internal jugular venous access for CVP or inotropic agents

2. Contraindications:
   a. Prior groin surgery (relative)
   b. Patient must maintain bedrest while the catheter is in place.

3. Anesthesia:

   1% lidocaine

4. Equipment:

   a. Sterile prep solution
   b. Sterile gloves and towels
   c. 25 gauge needle
   d. 5 mL syringes(2)
   e. Appropriate catheters and dilator
   f. IV tubing and flush
   g. 18 gauge insertion needle (5 cm long)
   h. .035 "J" wire
   i. Sterile dressings
   j. Safety razor
   k. Scalpel
   l. 2–0 silk suture

5. Positioning:

   Supine

6. Technique:

   a. Shave, sterile prep, and drape left or right groin area.
   b. Palpate the femoral pulse at the midpoint along an imagi-
      nary line between the anterior superior iliac spine and the
      symphysis pubis. The femoral vein runs parallel and imme-
      diately *medial* to the artery (Fig. 2.11).
   c. Administer anesthetic with 25 gauge needle into the skin
      and subcutaneous area 1 cm caudal and 1 cm lateral to the
      palpated pulse above.
   d. Palpate the femoral pulse and gently retract the artery later-
      ally.
   e. Using the 18 gauge insertion needle with a 5 mL syringe,
      puncture the anesthetized skin and advance the needle
      while aspirating cranially at a 45° angle to the skin, parallel
      to the pulse. There is *less risk with being medial* to the vein
      than lateral (Figs. 2.12 and 2.13).
   f. *If no venous blood return after 5 cm,* slow withdraw needle
      while aspirating. If still no return, redirect the needle
      through the same puncture site aiming cranial and gradu-
      ally 1–3 cm more lateral toward the artery.

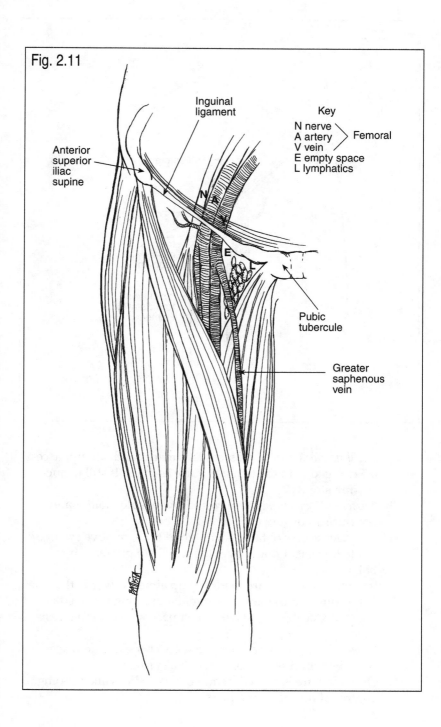

Fig. 2.11

Inguinal ligament

Key

N nerve
A artery
V vein   } Femoral
E empty space
L lymphatics

Anterior superior iliac supine

Pubic tubercule

Greater saphenous vein

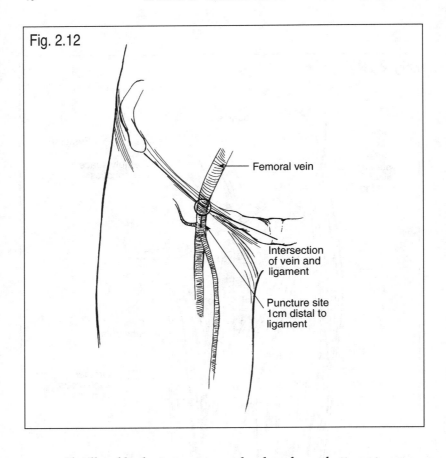

Fig. 2.12

Femoral vein

Intersection
of vein and
ligament

Puncture site
1cm distal to
ligament

g. *If still no blood return,* reassess landmarks and attempt access
0.5 cm medial to the femoral pulse as in (e). If still unsuccessful, stop.

h. *If arterial blood encountered,* withdraw needle, hold manual
pressure according to Section I.C.7 below.

i. If venous access obtained with good flow, remove syringe
while keeping a finger over the needle to prevent air embolism.

j. Introduce the "J" wire, with the tip aimed towards the
heart, through the needle while maintaining the needle in
the same location. The wire must pass with minimal resistance.

k. If resistance is met, remove the wire, check needle placement by withdrawing blood with a syringe.

l. Once the wire is passed, remove the needle while keeping
control of the wire *at all times.*

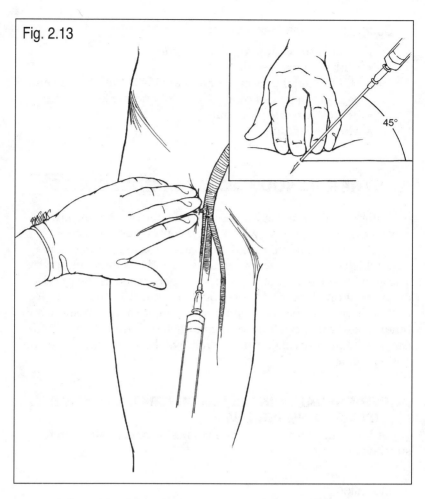

Fig. 2.13

45°

m. Enlarge the puncture site with a sterile scalpel.

n. Introduce the dilator over the wire 3–4 cm to *dilate the subcutaneous tissues only while keeping control of the wire.* Advancing the dilator the entire length can lacerate the femoral vein and is *not* recommended.

o. Remove the dilator and introduce the central venous catheter over the wire to the length of *15 cm.*

p. Remove the wire, aspirate blood from all ports to confirm venous placement, and then flush with sterile saline. Suture the catheter to the skin with silk suture. Dress the skin with a sterile dressing.

q. Patient must maintain bedrest until the catheter is removed.

7. Complications and Management:

a. Femoral artery puncture/hematoma
- Withdraw the needle.
- Hold manual pressure for at least 15–25 minutes. A sand-bag is then placed over the site for another 30 minutes.
- Bedrest for at least 4 hours.
- Monitor leg pulses.

II. OTHER VENOUS ACCESS PROCEDURES

Other forms of venous access include peripherally inserted central catheters (PICCs), which allow central venous access through a peripheral vein, and surgical access in emergent situation, which consists of venous cutdowns and intraosseous access. These procedures are not as commonly performed as the previously mentioned methods of venous access. In addition, included in this chapter is a protocol on removal of Hickman, Groshon, and other long-term indwelling venous catheters. Surgical house officers are frequently called upon to remove these devices in the outpatient clinics.

A. PERIPHERALLY INSERTED CENTRAL CATHETER (PICC), LONG ARM IV

A long, thin catheter inserted via basilic or cephalic vein to subclavian vein.

1. Indications:

a. Long term intravenous access for drugs
b. TPN fluids
c. *Not* for CVP monitoring

2. Contraindications:

a. Lack of upper arm veins visible or palpable with tourniquet in place
b. Presence of phlebitis or cellulitis in arm

3. Anesthesia:

1% lidocaine without epinephrine

4. Equipment:

 a. Most PICC kits come with everything necessary, including Betadine swabs, alcohol swabs, sterile drapes, 3 mL syringe and 25 g needle, introducer [14 gauge IV catheter (some catheters require peel-away design)], Silastic catheter with guide wire, scissors, needle-holder, 3–0 silk suture on a curved cutting needle, suture wing, Betadine ointment, lint-free 4 × 4 gauze pads, tape measure.

 b. Equipment not contained in kits include sterile gloves, sterile saline or water to rinse gloves and catheter, injectable heparinized saline to flush catheter at completion of the procedure.

5. Positioning:

Patient should be sitting or reclining comfortably with arm abducted to about 45° to axis of body and externally rotated. Arm should be slightly dependent; elbow should be extended.

6. Technique:

 a. Place tourniquet.

 b. Identify vein, preferably in forearm that is continuous with basilic or cephalic vein (Fig. 2.14).

 c. Prep with alcohol, then Betadine a large area around the point of anticipated insertion.

 d. Place sterile drape.

 e. Have assistant rinse your gloves.

 f. Have assistant pour saline over catheter.

 g. Measure length to approximate SVC site from insertion site.

 h. Using small amount of lidocaine, infiltrate skin on either side of vein; allow lidocaine to take effect.

 i. At this point in the procedure, kits that have attached hub require that the catheter be trimmed prior to insertion. Trim from the end opposite the hub (i.e., the tip). Do not trim the tip of a Groshon catheter.

 j. Flush Silastic catheter before inserting it.

 k. Place 14 gauge introducer catheter into vein as if inserting a peripheral IV. At sight of flash of blood, remove needle from catheter and slightly advance plastic portion of introducer (Fig. 2.15).

 l. Insert Silastic catheter through plastic introducer catheter.

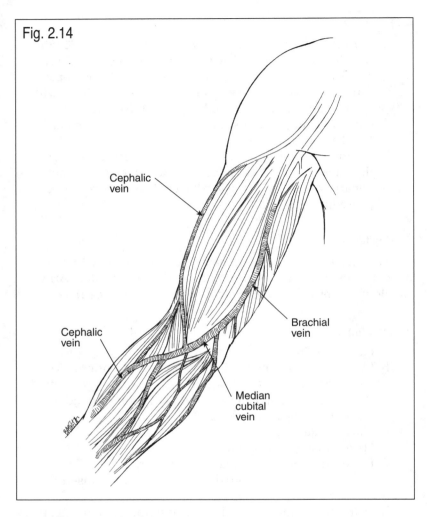

Fig. 2.14

Cephalic vein

Cephalic vein

Brachial vein

Median cubital vein

m. Remove tourniquet.
n. Advance Silastic catheter to premeasured length. (Some kits come with forceps to advance the catheter.)
o. Remove guide wire.
p. Remove or peel away plastic introducer catheter.
q. Trim end of Silastic catheter to manageable length, but only if it has a detachable hub.
r. Place attachable hub and hep-lock.
s. Place wings.
t. Suture catheter to the skin.
u. Withdraw blood.
v. Flush catheter.

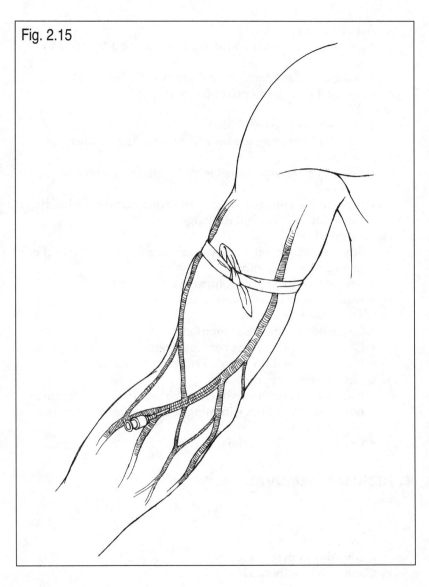

Fig. 2.15

w. Apply dressing.
x. Confirm placement with chest X-ray.

7. Complications and Management:

a. Bleeding
- Apply pressure at insertion site for at least 5 min.
- Treat coagulopathy and thrombocytopenia if necessary.

    b. Arrhythmia
- Usually secondary to the catheter being advanced too far
- Withdraw catheter until arrhythmia resolves.
- Medical management, if necessary

    c. Phlebitis
- Thought to be exacerbated by glove powder
- Prevent by rinsing gloves and minimizing handling of catheter.
- Treat by removing catheter and applying warm compresses.
- If purulent, culture and institute antibiotics accordingly. Consider incision and drainage.

    d. Line infection
- Suspected by positive blood cultures from the line and not from peripheral cultures.
- Remove catheter and culture tip.
- Institute appropriate antibiotics.

    e. Clotted catheter
- Be suspicious of intravenous clot.
- Obtain Doppler studies or venogram.
- If clot present, line removal recommended.

    f. Cracked or leaking catheter
- PICCs with attachable hub can be repaired by obtaining new attachable hub, trimming catheter slightly, and placing new hub.
- Other PICCs should be removed.

B. HICKMAN REMOVAL

1. Indications:

    a. Infected catheter
    b. Intractably clotted catheter
    c. Completion of therapy

2. Contraindications:

    a. Severe coagulopathy (PT or PTT >1.3X control)
    b. Continued need for therapy

3. Anesthesia:

    Local 1% lidocaine

4. Equipment:

a. Betadine prep solution
b. Sterile drapes
c. Sterile instruments
d. Hemostats
e. Scalpel with blade
f. Needle holder
g. 4–0 nylon suture

5. Positioning:

Supine

6. Technique:

a. Prep area where Hickman catheter emerges from skin, include catheter in prep.
b. Infiltrate area where catheter emerges with anesthesia; infiltrate tract up to and including cuff.
c. Apply gentle, steady pulling pressure to Hickman. Sometimes this is enough to dislodge the cuff from its surrounding fibrous tissue.
d. When cuff is close to skin incision, insert hemostat via tract to cuff site, and, using spreading technique bluntly, divide fibrous tissue (Fig. 2.16).
e. Occasionally it is necessary to enlarge the skin incision. Use the scalpel, taking care to avoid lacerating the catheter. If necessary, make an incision directly over the cuff and then use blunt dissection to free the cuff.
f. Once the cuff is freed from the fibrous tissue, gently and steadily pull the catheter from the tract.
g. Apply pressure to the subclavian or internal jugular area as tip of catheter exits the vein.
h. If skin incision is large, approximate edges with suture.
i. Apply dressing.

7. Complications and Management:

a. Air embolus
   • Unlikely with removal of tunneled catheter
   • If hemodynamically unstable (cardiac arrest), initiate ACLS and stat thoracic surgery consult.
   • If stable, place patient in left lateral decubitus and Trendelenburg position to trap air in right ventricle.

Fig. 2.16

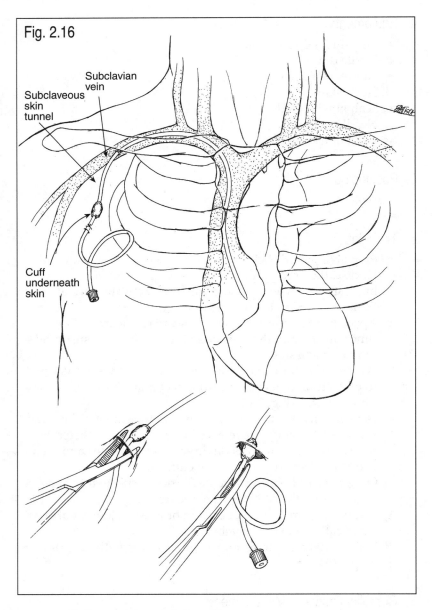

- Follow with serial chest X-rays.
- Air will eventually dissolve.
b. Bleeding
- Apply direct pressure for at least 5 min.
c. Catheter breakage
- If this occurs external to skin site, prevent air embolus by

clamping catheter proximal to break, and proceed to remove the catheter as above.
- If the break occurs underneath the skin and the end retracts through the tunnel, interventional radiology will need to retrieve the catheter.
- This is one of the most serious complications; avoid it by not pulling the catheter too hard and by keeping sharp instruments out of the tunnel.

C. GREATER SAPHENOUS VENOUS CUTDOWN

1. Indications:

Saphenous vein cutdown is performed when percutaneous access to the venous system cannot be gained. It can be used to gain lower extremity access for trauma but in recent years has been replaced by the percutaneous femoral vein approach. The referred site for saphenous vein cutdown is at the ankle. Although the saphenous vein can also be reached by a cutdown in the groin, this technique has very limited role as an elective bedside procedure.

2. Contraindications:

a. Coagulopathy (PT or PTT >1.3)
b. Vein thrombosis

3. Anesthesia:

Local 1% lidocaine

4. Equipment:

a. Tourniquet
b. Sterile prep solution
c. Sterile drape
d. Sterile gloves
e. 4 × 4 gauze pads
f. 3 mL syringe with 25 gauge needle
g. Scalpel
h. Hemostat
i. Fine scissors
j. IV catheter
k. Hep-lock cap

l. 3–0 silk ties
m. Topical antibiotic ointment

5. Positioning:

Patient should be in position comfortable for the operator, usually supine, with extremity of interest in dependent position.

6. Technique:

a. The greater saphenous vein is consistently located about 1 cm anterior and 1 cm superior to the medial malleolus (Fig. 2.17).

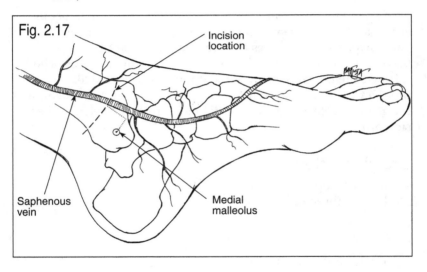

Fig. 2.17

Incision location

Saphenous vein

Medial malleolus

A tourniquet is not necessary for access to the vein.
b. Prep and drape area surrounding the ankle.
c. Infiltrate the skin over the vein with lidocaine using a 25 gauge needle.
d. Make a full thickness transverse incision through the anesthetized skin to a length of 2.5 cm.
e. Using a curved hemostat, identify the saphenous vein and gently dissect it free from the saphenous nerve, which is attached to the anterior wall of the vein. It is imperative that the saphenous nerve be identified to avoid injury and subsequent pain (Fig. 2.18).
f. Elevate and dissect the vein free from its bed for a distance of approximately 2 cm.

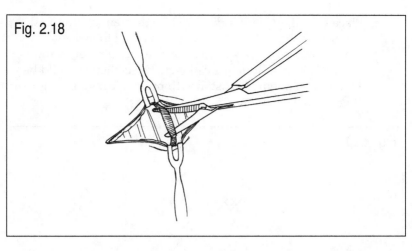

Fig. 2.18

g. Pass the silk sutures around the exposed vein proximally and distally.
h. Ligate the vein distally, leaving the suture in place for traction.
i. Make a small transverse venotomy and gently dilate the venotomy with the tip of the closed hemostat. A vein introducer may also be used (Fig. 2.19).

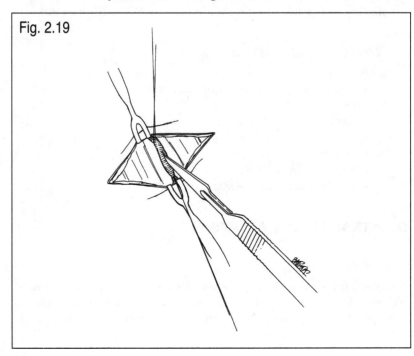

Fig. 2.19

   j. Place IV catheter either directly into the vein or after first
      tunnelling the catheter through skin distal to incision.
   k. Tie the proximal silk suture to secure the catheter, being
      careful not to occlude the catheter. The catheter should be
      inserted an adequate distance to prevent easy dislodgment
      (Fig. 2.20).

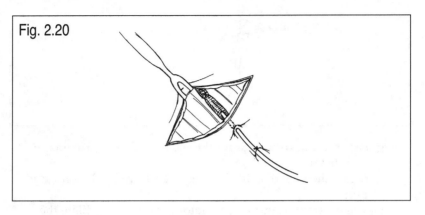

Fig. 2.20

   l. Begin intravenous infusion.
   m. Close wound with interrupted nylon suture.
   n. Apply a sterile dressing with topical antibiotic ointment.

7. Complications and Management:

   a. Bleeding
      • Apply pressure if bleeding occurs.
   b. Infection
      • Remove the catheter.
      • Use antibiotics, if necessary.
   c. Phlebitis
      • Remove the catheter.
      • Apply warm compresses.

D. INTRAOSSEOUS ACCESS

1. Indications:

   Need for emergency access, usually in a child less than 3 years
old, where other attempts at venous access have failed and time is
too short for a cutdown. The technique has been used in older chil-

dren and adults. Once intravascular volume has been replaced, other access can be obtained.

2. Contraindications:

a. As this is an emergency procedure and is to be used in the severely injured or critically ill patient, the only relative contraindication is injury to the extremity of interest.
b. Avoid placing the needle distal to a fracture site.

3. Anesthesia:

None

4. Equipment:

16 or 18 gauge bone marrow aspiration or intraosseous infusion needle

5. Positioning:

Supine

6. Technique:

a. Insert needle, bevel up, at 60–90° angle into the marrow of a long bone. The preferred site is the tibia 2–3 cm inferior to the tibial tuberosity. The inferior third of the femur can be used as an alternative (Fig. 2.21).
b. Aspiration of marrow confirms proper location. Other clues to proper position include firm upright position of needle in bone and easy infusion of 5–10 mL of fluid (Fig. 2.22).
c. Secure the needle with tape.

7. Complications and Management:

a. Infiltration
  • Remove and replace needle.
b. Cellulitis
  • Remove needle.
  • Treat cellulitis with antibiotics.
c. Osteomyelitis
  • Give appropriate long-term antibiotics.

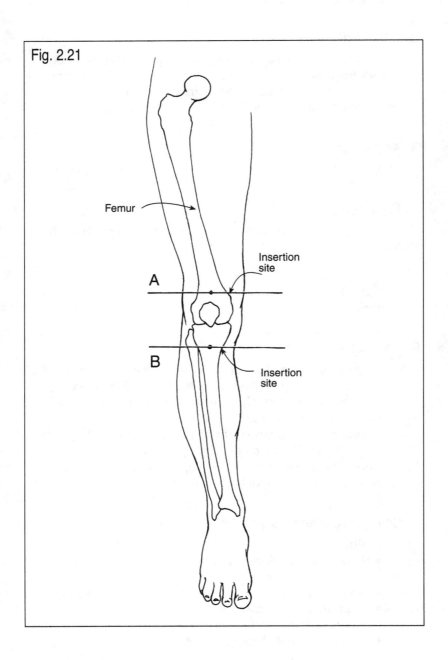

Fig. 2.21

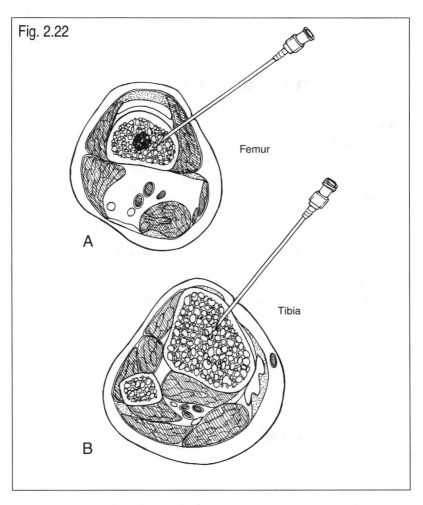

Fig. 2.22

Femur

A

Tibia

B

d. Compartment syndrome
  • Fasciotomy

III. ARTERIAL CANNULATION

Arterial lines permit continuous monitoring of heart rate and blood pressure necessary in ICU patients who are receiving inotropic agents or who are hemodynamically unstable. Intraoperative monitoring is also required with high risk patients. We prefer radial > femoral > dorsalis pedis > axillary. We recommend the quick catheters or IV angio catheters for the radial and dorsalis pedis arteries but the Seldinger technique for the femoral and axillary arteries.

A. RADIAL ARTERY CANNULATION

1. Indications:
   a. Continuous hemodynamic monitoring
   b. Frequent assessment of arterial blood gases

2. Contraindications:
Failed Allen's test
   a. Occlude both ulnar and radial arteries digitally and allow venous drainage to exsanguinate the hand (Fig. 2.23).
   b. Release the ulnar artery while keeping the radial compressed.
   c. If hand color does not return in <5 seconds, the patient has failed the Allen's test.

3. Anesthesia:
1% lidocaine

4. Equipment:
   a. Sterile prep solution
   b. Sterile gloves and towels
   c. 25 gauge needle
   d. Syringe
   e. 20 gauge angio catheter (2") or quick catheters
   f. 2–0 silk sutures
   g. Pressure bags with IV tubing
   h. Heparized flush system with sensor attachments for monitoring
   i. Sterile dressings
   j. Hand towel

5. Positioning:
Expose the ventral surface of the forearm, dorsiflex the wrist and place a rolled-up hand towel underneath the dorsal surface of the wrist. Secure the palm and forearm to an arm board.

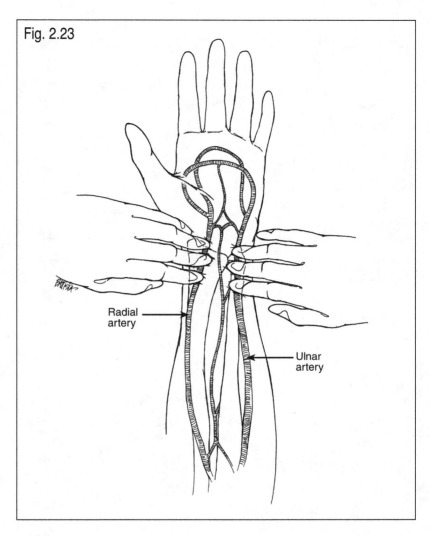

Fig. 2.23

Radial artery

Ulnar artery

6. Technique:
   a. Sterile prep and drape the ventral surface of the wrist.
   b. Palpate the radial pulse near the distal radius.
   c. Administer anesthetic with a 25 gauge needle into the skin above this point (Fig. 2.24).
   d. Using a 20 gauge angiocatheter with the bevel up, puncture the skin at a 45° angle to the skin. Advance the angio catheter toward the palpated pulse until blood return is seen in the hub of the needle (Fig. 2.25).
   e. *If no blood return in the hub,* withdraw the angio catheter

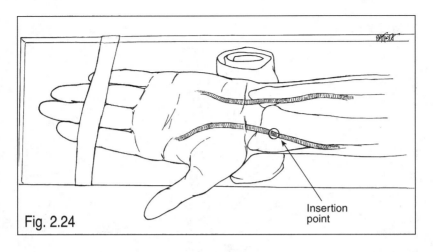

Insertion
point

Fig. 2.24

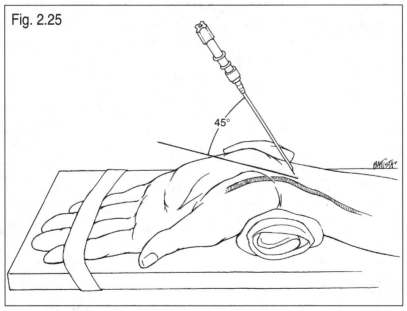

Fig. 2.25

45°

slowly and make another pass at a 60° angle toward the palpated pulse.

f. If *good blood return in the hub,* advance the angio catheter another 2 *mm* to ensure intraluminal placement of the catheter
portion of the angio catheter. *If you are using a quick catheter,*
this additional 2 mm is not necessary and the wire portion
of the system is then advanced into the artery at this point.

g. While maintaining a *firm hold on the needle* portion of the angio catheter, slowly advance the catheter portion into the artery.

h. Remove the needle and keep *digital compression* on the proximal radial artery to prevent excessive bleeding.

i. If there is *no bleeding*, then the catheter is not intraluminal. Withdraw the catheter slowly in case it has punctured the posterior wall. If still no blood, remove the catheter, hold digital pressure for *5 min*. Reassess landmarks and attempt again as in (d) to (h).

j. If successful, attach flush system and sensors to the monitor to assess arterial waveform.

k. Suture the catheter to the skin using the silk sutures and cover with a sterile dressing.

l. If unsuccessful after three attempts, stop and assess another site.

7. Complications and Management:
   a. Poor arterial waveform
      - Check all line connections and stopcocks.
      - Exclude extrinsic proximal arterial compression.
      - Check the position of the arm and wrist. The arm cannot be elevated and the wrist must be dorsiflexed.
      - If waveform and the blood return is poor, replace the catheter.
   b. Ischemic digits or thrombosis
      - Remove the catheter and closely monitor the digit.

B. DORSALIS PEDIS ARTERY CANNULATION

1. Indications:
   a. Continuous hemodynamic monitoring
   b. Frequent assessment of arterial blood gases

2. Contraindications:
   No palpable dorsalis artery

3. Anesthesia:
   1% lidocaine

4. Equipment:

a. Sterile prep solution
b. Sterile gloves and towels
c. 25 gauge needle
d. 5 mL syringe
e. 20 gauge angio catheter (2″) or quick catheters
f. 2–0 silk sutures
g. Pressure bags with IV tubing
h. Heparized flush system with sensor attachments for monitoring
i. Sterile dressings.

5. Positioning:

Expose the dorsal surface of the foot in neutral position.

6. Technique:

a. Sterile prep and drape dorsal surface of the foot.
b. Palpate the dorsalis pedis pulse lateral to the extensor hallucis longus at the level of the metatarsal-1st cuneiform joint (Fig. 2.26).
c. Administer anesthetic with a 25 gauge needle into the skin above this point.
d. Using a 20 gauge angio catheter with the bevel up, puncture the skin at a 45° angle to the skin. Advance the angio catheter toward the palpated pulse until blood return is seen in the hub of the needle (Fig. 2.27).
e. *If no blood return in the hub,* withdraw the angio catheter slowly and make another pass at a 60° angle toward the palpated pulse.
f. If *good blood return in the hub,* advance the angio catheter another 2 *mm* to ensure intraluminal placement of the catheter portion of the angio catheter. *If you are using a quick catheter,* this additional 2 mm is not necessary and the wire portion of the system is then advanced into the artery at this point.
g. While maintaining a *firm hold on the needle* portion of the angio catheter, slowly advance the catheter portion into the artery.
h. Remove the needle and keep *digital compression* proximally to prevent excessive bleeding.
i. If there is *no bleeding*, then the catheter is not intraluminal.

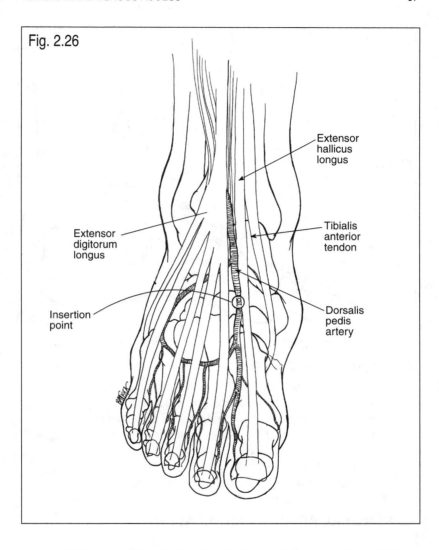

Fig. 2.26

Extensor hallicus longus

Extensor digitorum longus

Tibialis anterior tendon

Insertion point

Dorsalis pedis artery

Withdraw the catheter slowly in case it has punctured the posterior wall. If still no blood, remove the catheter, hold digital pressure for *15 min*. Reassess landmarks and attempt again as in (d) to (h).

j. If successful, attach flush system and sensors to the monitor to assess arterial waveform.

k. Suture the catheter to the skin using the silk sutures and cover with a sterile dressing.

l. If unsuccessful after three attempts, stop and assess another site.

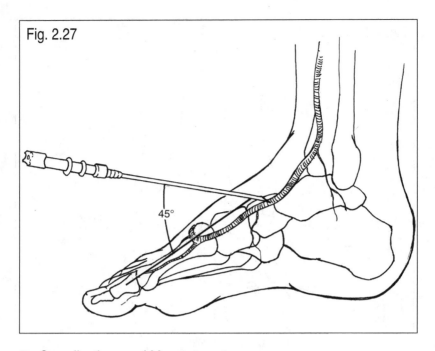

Fig. 2.27

45°

7. Complications and Management:

a. Poor arterial waveform
- Check all line connections and stopcocks.
- Exclude extrinsic proximal arterial compression.
- If waveform and the blood return is poor, replace the catheter.

b. Ischemic toes or thrombosis
- Remove the catheter and closely monitor the digit.

C. FEMORAL ARTERY CANNULATION

1. Indications:

a. Continuous hemodynamic monitoring
b. Frequent assessment of arterial blood gases
c. Access for arteriography studies
d. Intra-aortic balloon pump insertion (see Chapter 3)

2. Contraindications:

a. Iliac or femoral arterial vascular graft in place
b. Prior groin surgery (relative)
c. Patient must maintain bedrest while the catheter is in place.

3. Anesthesia:

1% lidocaine

4. Equipment:

a. Sterile prep solution
b. Sterile gloves and towels
c. 25 gauge needle
d. 5 mL syringes (2)
e. 16 gauge catheter (6")
f. 18 gauge insertion needle (5 cm long)
g. .035 "J" wire
h. Sterile dressings
i. Safety razor
j. 2–0 silk sutures
k. Pressure bags with IV tubing
l. Heparized flush system with sensor attachments for monitoring

5. Positioning:

Supine

6. Technique:

a. Shave, sterile prep, and drape left or right groin area
b. Palpate the femoral pulse at the midpoint along an imaginary line between the *anterior superior iliac spine* and the *symphysis pubis*. Palpate its course 1–2 cm distally.
c. Administer anesthetic with 25 gauge needle into the skin and subcutaneous area along the course of the artery palpated above (Fig. 2.28).
d. Using the 18 gauge insertion needle with a 5 mL syringe, puncture the skin at Point A and advance the needle while aspirating cranially at a 45° angle to the skin toward the pulse (Fig. 2.29 and 2.30).
e. *If no arterial blood return after 5 cm,* slow withdraw needle while aspirating. If still no return, redirect again toward to palpated pulse.
f. *If still no blood return,* reassess landmarks and attempt access 1 cm more proximal along the course of the artery as in (d). If still unsuccessful, stop.
g. *If venous blood encountered,* withdraw needle, hold manual pressure according to Section III.C.7 below.

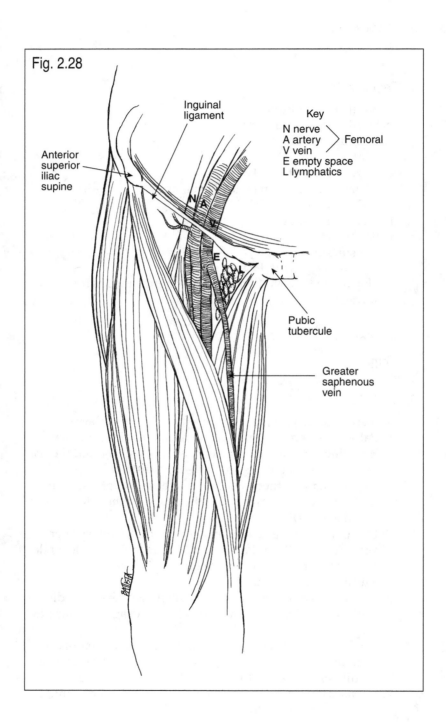

Fig. 2.28

Inguinal ligament

Anterior superior iliac supine

Key

N nerve
A artery
V vein   Femoral
E empty space
L lymphatics

Pubic tubercule

Greater saphenous vein

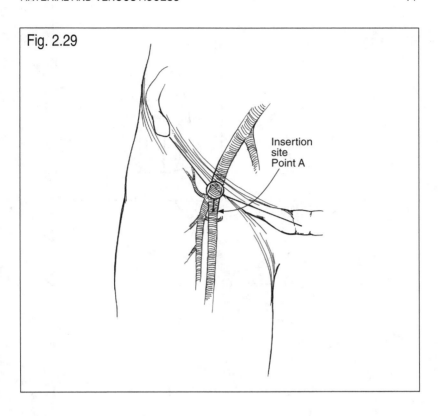

Fig. 2.29

Insertion
site
Point A

h. If arterial access obtained, remove the syringe while keeping
a finger over the needle to prevent excessive bleeding.
i. Introduce the "J" wire, with the tip aimed towards the heart,
through the needle while maintaining the needle in the
same location (Seldinger technique). The wire must pass
with minimal resistance.
j. If resistance is met, remove the wire and check needle placement by withdrawing blood with a syringe.
k. Once the wire is passed, remove the needle while keeping
control of the wire *at all times*.
l. Enlarge the puncture site carefully with a sterile scalpel.
m.Introduce the central venous catheter over the wire.
n. Remove the wire and attach flush system and sensors to the
monitor to assess arterial waveform. Suture the catheter to
the skin with silk suture. Dress the skin with a sterile dressing.
o. Patient must maintain bedrest until the catheter is removed.

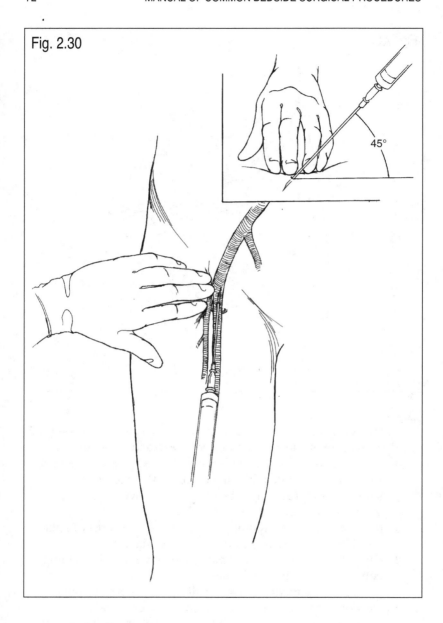

Fig. 2.30

7. Complications and Management:

a. Femoral vein puncture
- Withdraw the needle.
- Hold manual pressure for at least 10 minutes.

b. Thrombosis
- Remove the catheter.

- Closely monitor leg pulses and observe for distal emboli.
  c. Hematoma
    - Remove the catheter.
    - Hold manual pressure for at least 15–25 minutes. A sandbag is then placed over the site for another 30 minutes.
    - Bedrest for at least 4 hours.
    - Monitor leg pulses.

D. AXILLARY ARTERY CANNULATION

1. Indications:
   a. Continuous hemodynamic monitoring
   b. Frequent assessment of arterial blood gases
   c. Access for arteriography studies

2. Contraindications:
   a. Unable to abduct arm
   b. Poor distal peripheral pulses

3. Anesthesia:
   1% lidocaine

4. Equipment:
   a. Sterile prep solution
   b. Sterile gloves and towels
   c. 25 gauge needle
   d. 5 mL syringes (2)
   e. 16 gauge catheter (6″)
   f. 18 gauge insertion needle (5 cm long)
   g. .035 "J" wire
   h. Sterile dressings
   i. Safety razor
   j. 2–0 silk sutures
   k. Pressure bags with IV tubing
   l. Heparized flush system with sensor attachments for monitoring

5. Positioning:
   Supine with the shoulder externally rotated and the arm fully abducted

6. Technique:

a. Shave, sterile prep, and drape axilla.

b. Palpate the axillary pulse as proximal as possible inferior to the pectoralis major (Fig 2.31).

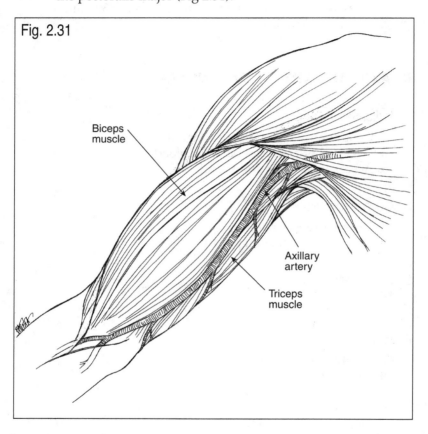

Fig. 2.31

Biceps muscle

Axillary artery

Triceps muscle

c. Administer anesthetic with 25 gauge needle into the skin and subcutaneous area along the course of the artery palpated above.

d. Using the 18 gauge insertion needle with a 5 mL syringe, puncture the anesthetized skin and advance the needle while aspirating at a 45° angle to the skin toward the pulse (Fig. 2.32).

e. *If no arterial blood return after 5 cm,* slow withdraw needle while aspirating. If still no return, redirect again toward to palpated pulse.

f. *If still no blood return,* reassess landmarks and attempt access 1 cm more distal along the course of the artery as in (d). If still unsuccessful, stop.

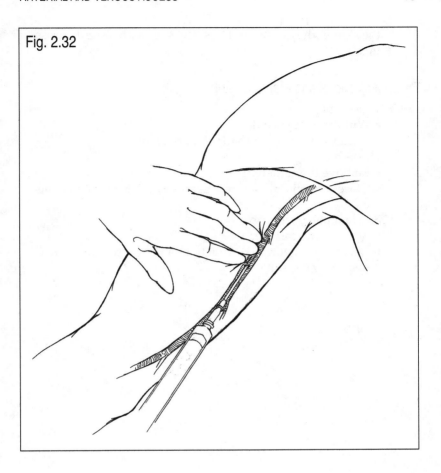

Fig. 2.32

g. *If venous blood encountered,* withdraw needle, hold manual pressure according to Section III.D.7 below.

h. If arterial access obtained, remove the syringe while keeping a finger over the needle to prevent excessive bleeding.

i. Introduce the "J" wire, with the tip aimed towards the heart, through the needle while maintaining the needle in the same location. The wire must pass with minimal resistance.

j. If resistance is met, remove the wire and check needle placement by withdrawing blood with a syringe.

k. Once the wire is passed, remove the needle while keeping control of the wire *at all times*.

l. Enlarge the puncture site carefully with a sterile scalpel.

m. Introduce the central venous catheter over the wire.

n. Remove the wire and attach flush system and sensors to the monitor to assess arterial waveform. Suture the catheter to the skin with silk suture. Dress the skin with a sterile dressing.

7. Complications and Management:

a. Venous puncture
  • Withdraw the needle.
  • Hold manual pressure for at least 10 minutes.
b. Thrombosis
  • Remove the catheter.
  • Closely monitor distal pulses and watch for ischemic digits.
c. Brachial plexus injury
  • Remove the catheter.
  • Observe for neurologic function. If no improvement, neurosurgery consult.

CHAPTER 3

CARDIOTHORACIC PROCEDURES

Authors: Elizabeth A. Davis, M.D., Peter J. Gruber, M.D., Ph.D., Paul P. Lin, M.D., and Herbert Chen, M.D.

CARDIOTHORACIC PROCEDURES

I. CARDIAC PROCEDURES

Bedside cardiac procedures can be life-saving maneuvers in cardiac surgery patients as well as other medical and surgical patients. Several of the following procedures should be routine to all houseofficers. However, surgical housestaff should especially be familiar with the more invasive techniques such as pericardiocentesis, pulmonary artery catheter placement, and intra-aortic balloon pump use.

A. DEFIBRILLATION/CARDIOVERSION

1. Indications:
    a. For defibrillation
        - Ventricular fibrillation (VF)
        - Pulseless ventricular tachycardia (VT)
    b. Cardioversion
        - Any hemodynamically unstable tachyarrhythmia other than VF or pulseless VT

2. Contraindications:
    None

3. Anesthesia:

If time and the patient's blood pressure permit, may give a sedative (diazepam, midazolam, ketamine) with or without an analgesic agent (fentanyl, morphine). See Appendix B.

4. Equipment:

a. Electrode gel
b. Defibrillator
c. EKG machine

5. Positioning:

a. The patient should be supine away from water or metal surfaces.
b. Expose the chest fully (remove any transdermal patches).

6. Technique:

a. Apply gel to hand-held paddles or use adhesive electrode pads.
b. Turn on machine. Set to defibrillate (asynchronous) for VF or VT or cardiovert (synchronous) for all other arrhythmias. See chart below.

electroconversion	defibrillate	cardiovert
mode	asynchronous	synchronous
arrhythmia	VT or VF	other unstable arrhythmias
1st shock	200 J	50 or 100 J
2nd shock	300 J	200 J
3rd shock	360 J	300 or 360 J

c. Set machine to appropriate energy level. The first shock should be 200 J for defibrillation and 50 or 100 J for electroconversion.
d. Charge the capacitor.
e. Place electrodes on chest. There are two acceptable placements:
  • One electrode to the right of the upper sternum and the other over the apex of the heart to the left of the nipple in the midaxillary line (Fig. 3.1)
  • One electrode anteriorly over the left precordium (A) and the other posteriorly beneath the left scapula (B) (Fig. 3.2)

Avoid positioning electrodes over pacemakers.

f. Apply 25 pounds of pressure to hand-held paddles. An-

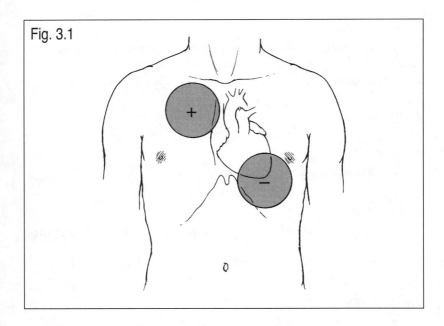

Fig. 3.1

nounce that defibrillation/cardioversion is about to occur
and loudly state "All clear!"
g. *Insure that no person is in contact with the patient or bed.*
h. Deliver an electric shock by pressing both discharge buttons
simultaneously.
i. If no response by the patient, repeat shock at next level.

7. Complications and Management:

a. Inadvertent shock to bystanders
   - Usually only results in temporary discomfort of the recipient
   - The best treatment is prevention.
b. Temporary or permanent pacemaker malfunction
   - After the patient is successfully resuscitated and hemodynamically stable, it may be necessary to interrogate and/or reset the pacemaker.
   - Place a transcutaneous pacer or insert a temporary transvenous pacer if needed (see Section C).
c. Cutaneous burns
   - Usually only first degree burns, but can extend deeper.
   - Treat according to depth of burn.

Fig. 3.2

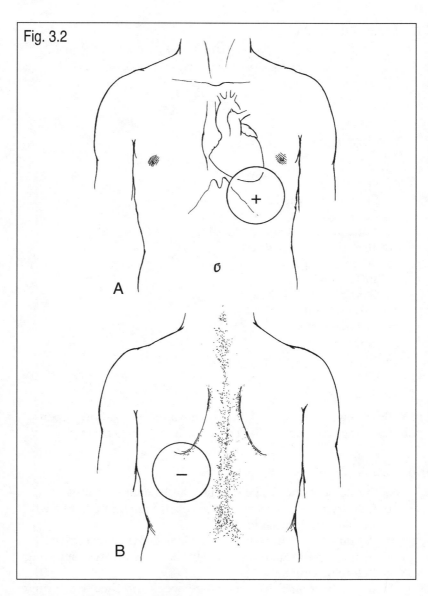

B. PERICARDIOCENTESIS

1. Indications:

   a. Relief of cardiac tamponade
   b. Diagnostic sampling of pericarditis or pericardial effusion

2. Contraindications:

   a. Coagulopathy (platelets <50k, PT or PTT > 1.3 × control)
   b. Post-cardiac bypass surgery because of risk of injury to
      grafts

3. Anesthesia:

   1% lidocaine

4. Equipment:

   a. Sterile prep solution
   b. Sterile gloves and towels
   c. Long 3" 16 or 18 gauge needle
   d. 16 gauge Teflon catheter
   e. 30 mL syringe
   f. EKG monitor
   g. Sterile alligator connector
   h. 0.035 "J" wire
   i. 2–0 nylon suture
   j. Safety razor
   k. Scalpel and blade

5. Positioning:

   Supine with the head of the bed elevated 30° to allow dependent pooling of blood or effusion to the area to be aspirated

6. Technique:

   a. Sterile prep and drape the chest and subxiphoid area.
   b. Identify the entry site of the needle 0.5 cm immediately left
      of the xiphoid tip (Fig. 3.3).
   c. Administer 1% lidocaine with a 25 gauge needle into the
      skin and subcutaneous tissue in this area, always aspirating
      before injecting.
   d. Insert the long 3" 16 or 18 gauge needle attached to a syringe
      through the anesthetized skin 0.5 cm immediately left of the
      xiphoid tip.
   e. Attach a precordial limb lead of the EKG machine to the
      needle with an alligator clip for monitoring.
   f. Advance the needle through the skin at a 45° *angle to the tho-
      rax* underneath the sternum and directed posteriorly, aiming
      toward the left shoulder. Apply continuous aspiration (Fig. 3.4).

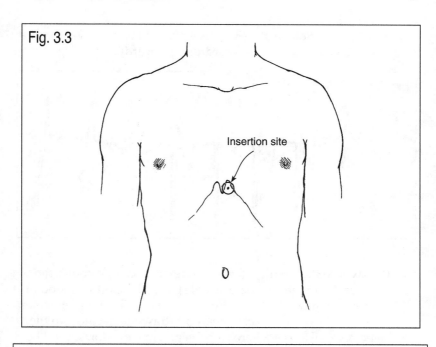

Fig. 3.3

Insertion site

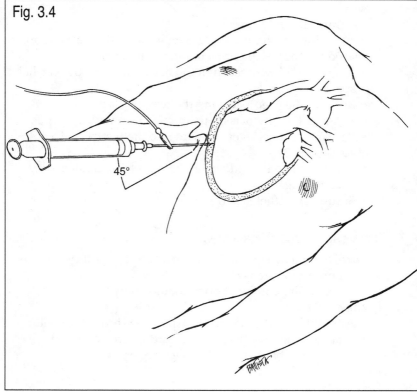

Fig. 3.4

45°

g. *Negative deflection of the QRS complex* will be seen when contact is made with the epicardium (pericardial sac) (Fig. 3.5).

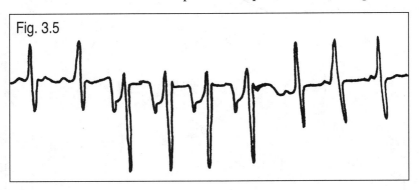

Fig. 3.5

h. Advance the needle a few centimeters further through the epicardium into the pericardial space. Nonclotting blood or effusion may be encountered. *ST segment* elevation indicates contact with the *myocardium*. Withdraw the needle into the pericardial space where no ST segment elevation should be seen.
i. Aspirate all fluid present.
j. For continuous drainage a 16 gauge soft Teflon catheter may placed via the Seldinger technique as follows.
   • Insert the "J" wire through the needle into the pericardial space.
   • Remove the needle leaving the wire in place.
   • Enlarge the skin incision to about 0.3 cm with a scalpel.
   • Pass the catheter over the wire into the pericardial space (Fig. 3.6).
   • Remove the wire and attach the catheter to a *closed system drainage* bag.
   • Suture the catheter to the skin.

7. Complications and Management:

a. Cardiac puncture or laceration of a coronary artery
   • Monitor vital signs closely.
   • May require emergent open thoracotomy.
b. Air embolus
   • Attempt to withdraw air by aspirating through catheter.
   • If hemodynamically unstable (cardiac arrest), initiate ACLS and obtain a stat thoracic surgery consult.

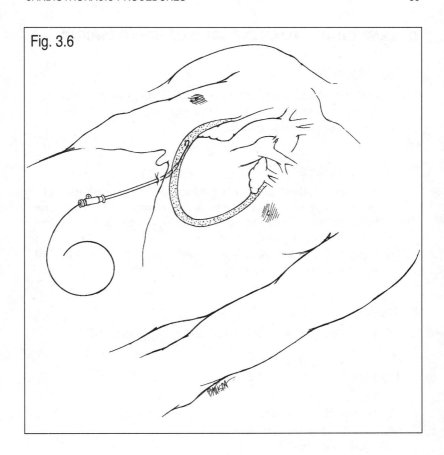

Fig. 3.6

- If stable, position patient in left lateral decubitus and Trendelenburg position to trap air in right ventricle. Chest X-ray in this position can demonstrate significant air and be used for follow-up.
- Air will eventually dissolve.
c. Cardiac arrhythmias
- Withdraw needle if hemodynamically significant.
- May require appropriate pharmacotherapy or electroconversion.
d. Hemothorax or pneumothorax
- Monitor with serial chest X-rays
- If significant, tube thoracostomy (see Section II).
e. Infection
- Catheter should only be left in place for 48 hours.
- Treat with appropriate antibiotics.

C. TEMPORARY TRANSVENOUS CARDIAC PACING

1. Indications:
   a. Perioperative management of cardiac surgery patients
   b. Short-term treatment of arrhythmias and heart block
   c. Emergency cardiac pacing

2. Contraindications:
   a. Severe hypothermia. Bradycardia may be physiologic in hypothermic patients. As the patient's temperature drops, the heart becomes more irritable creating potential for fibrillation with attempted pacing.
   b. Cardiac arrest for more than 20 minutes. Low likelihood of successful resuscitation.

3. Anesthesia:
   A sedative agent and an analgesic (see Appendix B)

4. Equipment:
   a. Sterile prep solution
   b. Sterile gloves and towels
   c. 22 and 25 gauge needles
   d. 5 mL syringes (2)
   e. Shoulder roll towels
   f. Appropriate catheters (cordis and sheath) and dilator
   g. IV tubing and flush
   h. 18 gauge insertion needle (5–8 cm long)
   i. .035 "J" wire
   j. Sterile dressings
   k. Scalpel
   l. 2–0 silk suture
   m. Pacer
   n. EKG monitor
   o. Alligator clips

5. Positioning:
   Supine

6. Technique:

    a. Insert a cordis central venous catheter into internal jugular vein or subclavian vein per Chapter 2, Section I.

    b. Attach EKG lead "V" with the alligator clip to the distal lead of the pacing catheter.

    c. *Gently* advance the pacing catheter through the cordis into the internal jugular or subclavian vein using sterile technique (Fig. 3.7).

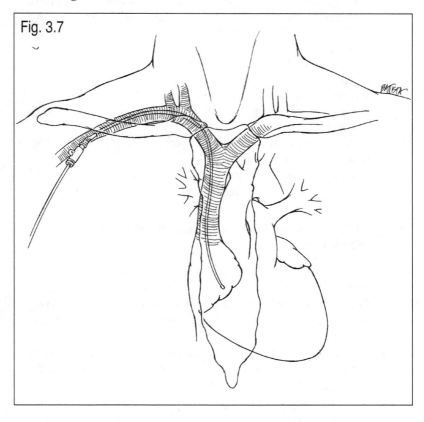

Fig. 3.7

    d. As the tip of the catheter enters the right atrium, the P wave on the EKG monitor will become very large.

    e. As the tip of the catheter enters the right ventricle, the QRS complex on the EKG monitor will enlarge.

    f. ST segment elevation indicates desired placement of the pacing catheter tip against the right ventricular wall.

    g. Secure the catheter in this position by suturing it to the cordis and to the skin.

    h. Attach the pacing leads to the pulse generator and initiate
       pacing.

7. Complications and Management:

    a. Lead-electrode catheter displacement
- Usually manifest by loss of capture or sensing
- Obtain chest X-ray.
- When displacement is recognized, the catheter should be immediately repositioned or removed and a new pacing catheter inserted if needed.

    b. Infection
- Remove catheter and culture.
- Start systemic antibiotics.
- If pacing is necessary insert a new catheter at a new site.

    c. Thrombophlebitis
- Remove the catheter and reinsert at a new site.

    d. Diaphragmatic stimulation
- May compromise ventilation.
- Reposition the catheter tip to minimize stimulation.

D. PULMONARY ARTERY (PA) OR SWAN GANZ CATHETER

1. Indications:

    a. Evaluation of therapeutic interventions (fluid, vasoactive agents, assisted circulation and ventilation, emergency cardiac pacing)

    b. Monitoring hemodynamic parameters in patients with low cardiac output syndromes or severe congestive heart failure (especially after open heart surgery)

2. Contraindications:

    a. Vein thrombosis
    b. Coagulopathy (PT or PTT > 1.3 ratio, platelets < 20K)
    c. Untreated ongoing sepsis
    d. Severe pulmonary hypertension

3. Anesthesia:

    1% lidocaine

4. Equipment:

a. Sterile prep solution
b. Sterile gloves and towels
c. 22 and 25 gauge needles
d. 5 mL syringes (2)
e. Shoulder roll towels
f. Cordis catheter and dilator (Cordis introducer kit)
g. IV tubing and flush
h. 18 gauge insertion needle (5–8 cm long)
i. .035 "J" wire
j. Sterile dressings
k. Scalpel handle and #10 blade
l. 2–0 silk suture
m. Swan Ganz catheter kit

5. Positioning:

Supine in Trendelenburg

6. Technique:

a. A cordis sheath introducer should be inserted first into one of the *IJ or subclavian veins* using sterile Seldinger technique. PA catheters generally should only be placed through the IJ or subclavian vein. Only in dire situations should a PA catheter be placed in the groin due to risk of infection. See Chapter 2, Section I.
b. When the insertion site is prepped and draped, the catheter should be removed from its container and tested.
c. Test the balloon by inflating and deflating it with the appropriate volume of air (usually 1.5 mL). Look for air leaks (Fig. 3.8).
d. In succession, flush each of the three ports (proximal, distal, PA) with sterile saline. Connect the pressure monitoring line to the transducer.
e. Place a protective plastic sheath over the catheter.
f. Pass a catheter (with the balloon deflated) into the subclavian or internal jugular vein through the cordis.
g. When the catheter has been inserted a distance of 20 cm (according to the ruler on the catheter itself), inflate the balloon with 1.5 mL of air. *Do not overinflate the balloon.*
h. Gently advance the catheter with the balloon inflated into the SVC or right atrium. A CVP waveform should appear on the monitor.

Fig. 3.8

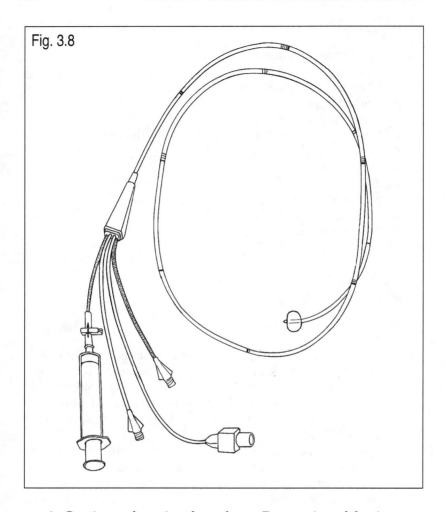

i. Continue advancing the catheter. Progression of the tip through the right ventricle (RV) (40 cm) and pulmonary artery (PA) (50 cm) will be manifest by the appropriate waveforms (Figs. 3.9 and 3.10).

j. If the RV or PA tracing has not appeared after 60–70 cm, *deflate the balloon,* withdraw the catheter to 20 cm, inflate the balloon, and attempt another insertion. *Any time the catheter needs to be withdrawn the balloon should be deflated. Any time the catheter needs to be advanced the balloon should be inflated.*

k. When the catheter reaches a wedged position, the waveform will dampen.

l. When this occurs, the balloon should be deflated and a PA

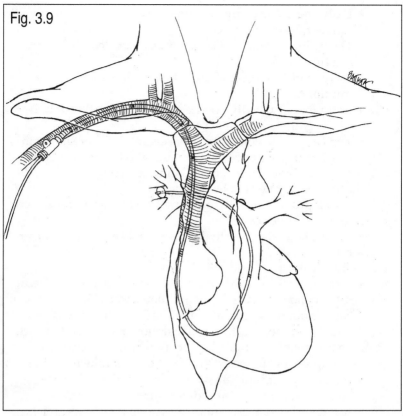

Fig. 3.9

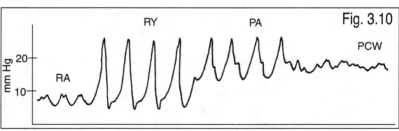

Fig. 3.10

tracing should appear. Leave the balloon deflated when the
desired position is achieved.

7. Complications and Management:

   a. Pulmonary infarction from "overwedging" the catheter
- Such a complication can be avoided by pulling the
catheter back when the pulmonary artery phasic pressures
become dampened on the monitor.

- Daily chest X-rays are recommended to monitor the catheter tip position.
- The balloon should *not be inflated for more than 1–2 minutes* at a time.
- Oxygenation and ventilatory support if needed

b. Arrhythmias
  - Arrhythmias usually occur as the tip passes through the right ventricle.
  - Typically these consist of only several PVCs or short runs of VT that cease once the tip enters the PA. If, however, they persist and are hemodynamically compromising, the catheter may need to be removed.
  - Check proper position to ensure the catheter is not curled in the right ventricle.
  - Medical therapy if arrhythmias do not stop after catheter removal.

c. Balloon rupture
  - Leakage of 0.8–1.5 mL of air into the circulation can occur if the balloon breaks. In the pulmonary circulation this can cause pulmonary infarction. If the foramen ovale is patent and the balloon ruptures on insertion into the right heart, an air embolus could enter a coronary or cerebral artery with potential myocardial infarction or stroke resulting.
  - If hemodynamically unstable (cardiac arrest), initiate ACLS and obtain a stat thoracic surgery consult.
  - If stable, position patient in left lateral decubitus and Trendelenburg position to trap air in right ventricle. Chest X-ray in this position can demonstrate significant air and be used for follow-up.
  - Air will eventually dissolve.

d. Pneumothorax
  - If a tension pneumothorax is suspected, decompress with 16 gauge angiocatheter placed into 2nd intercostal mid-clavicular space.
  - If <10%, 100% oxygen and serial 4-hour chest X-rays.
  - If >10%, tube thoracostomy (see Section II.B).

e. Rupture of the pulmonary artery
  - Pulmonary artery rupture is fatal. It can be prevented by avoiding "overwedging."
  - Emergent cardiac surgery

f. Knotting of the catheter
  - The catheter may become coiled during advancement or withdrawal. If any resistance is met during positioning of

the catheter, the attempt should be aborted and a chest X-ray obtained to verify position.
- Fluoroscopy may be needed to uncoil the catheter.
g. Infection
  - The incidence of infection is increased by frequent catheter manipulation and leaving the catheter in place for more than 3 days.
  - Treatment requires removal of the catheter and administration of antibiotics.

E. INTRA-AORTIC BALLOON PUMP (IABP)

1. Indications:
a. Cardiogenic shock
b. Refractory left ventricular failure
c. Mechanical complications of acute MI (VSD, papillary muscle dysfunction or rupture)
d. Unstable angina refractory to medical management
e. Ischemia induced ventricular arrhythmias
f. Support during PTCA
g. Weaning from cardiopulmonary bypass
h. Bridge to transplantation

2. Contraindications:
a. Irreversible brain damage
b. Chronic end-stage heart disease
c. Dissecting thoracic or aortic aneurysm
d. Aortic insufficiency
e. Severe peripheral vascular disease

3. Anesthesia:
1% lidocaine

4. Equipment:
a. Sterile prep solution
b. Sterile gloves and towels
c. Angiographic needle*
d. Guide wire*
e. Scalpel handle and #10 blade
f. Arterial dilator*

   g. Tissue clamp
   h. Sterile saline
   i. Lubricant
   j. IABP catheter*
   k. Arterial pressure monitoring system
   l. IABP system*
   m. 2–0 silk suture
   n. Transparent sterile tape or dressing
   o. Safety razor
   p. 0.035 "J" wire
   q. Whenever possible, fluoroscopy should be used during insertion to insure proper balloon placement.
   (*contained in most IABP insertion kits)

5. Positioning:

Supine in a monitored setting.

6. Technique—Insertion:

   a. Shave, sterile prep, and drape left or right groin area.
   b. Palpate the femoral pulse at the midpoint along an imaginary line between the *anterior superior iliac spine* and the *symphysis pubis*. Palpate its course 1–2 cm distally (Fig. 3.11).
   c. Administer anesthetic with 25 gauge needle into the skin and subcutaneous tissue along the course of the artery palpated above.
   d. Using the 18 gauge insertion needle with a 5 mL syringe, puncture the skin at point A and advance the needle while aspirating cranially at a 45° angle to the skin toward the pulse (Fig. 3.12).
   e. *If no arterial blood return after 5 cm,* slowly withdraw needle while aspirating. If still no return, redirect again toward the palpated pulse.
   f. *If still no blood return,* reassess landmarks and attempt access 1 cm more proximal along the course of the artery as in (d). If still unsuccessful, stop.
   g. *If venous blood encountered,* withdraw needle, hold manual pressure.
   h. If arterial access obtained, remove the syringe while keeping a finger over the needle to prevent excessive bleeding.
   i. Introduce the "J" wire, with the tip aimed towards the heart, through the needle while maintaining the needle in

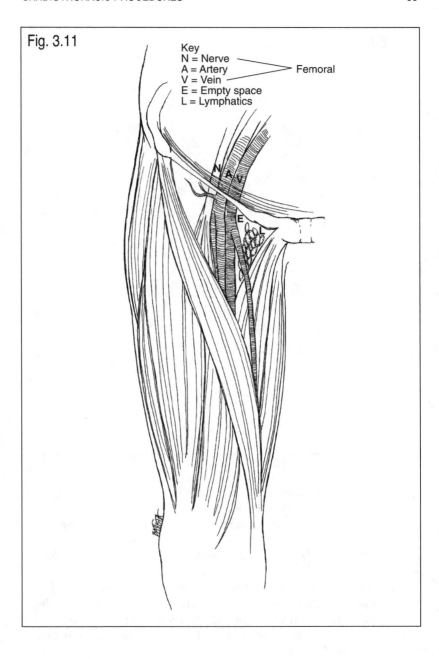

Fig. 3.11

Key
N = Nerve
A = Artery
V = Vein
E = Empty space
L = Lymphatics

Femoral

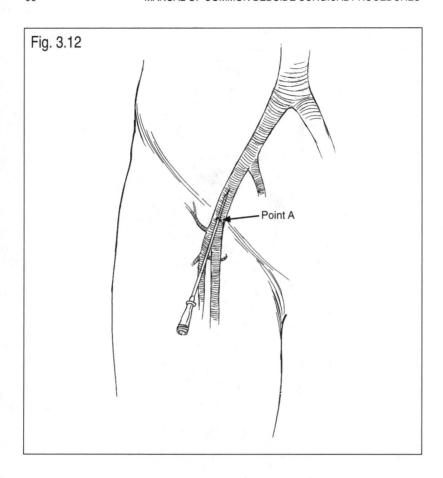

Fig. 3.12

Point A

the same location (Seldinger technique). The wire must pass with minimal resistance.

j. If resistance is met, remove the wire and check needle placement by withdrawing blood with a syringe.

k. Once the wire is passed, remove the needle while keeping control of the wire *at all times.*

l. Enlarge the puncture site carefully with a sterile scalpel.

m. Place the dilator over the "J" wire. Advance it through the skin into the arterial lumen. Then remove the dilator.

n. Using the tissue clamp, spread the subcutaneous tissue at the insertion site.

o. Remove the IABP catheter from the kit and lubricate it with sterile saline.

p. Remove the inner stylet (Fig. 3.13).

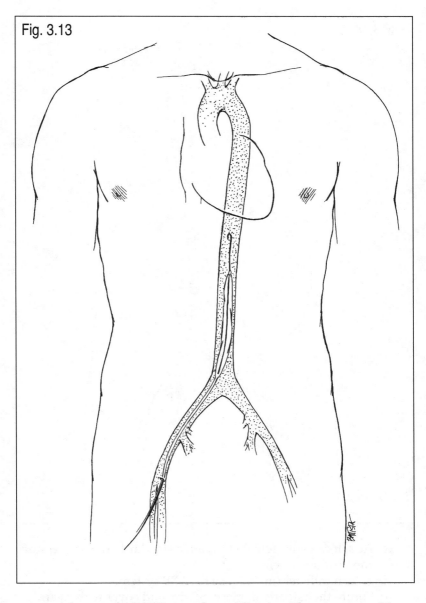

Fig. 3.13

q. Advance the IABP over the guide wire. The proper position of the catheter is with the balloon tip approximately 2 cm distal to the left subclavian artery in the descending thoracic aorta (Fig. 3.14).

r. Remove the guide wire and confirm intra-arterial placement by aspirating blood.

Fig. 3.14

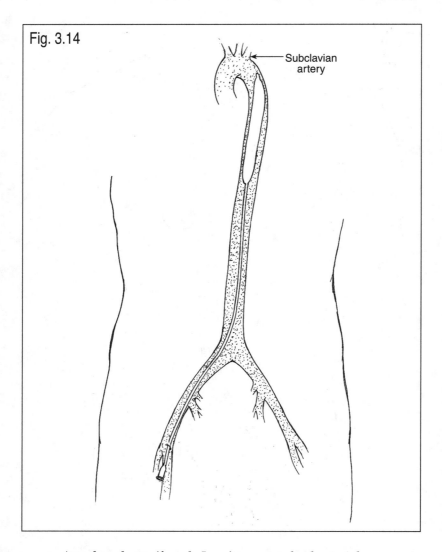

Subclavian artery

s. Attach catheter (female Luer) to a standard arterial pressure monitoring system.

t. Attach catheter (male Luer) to IABP system.

u. Suture the catheter in place. Secure and cover with clear sterile tape.

v. Obtain portable chest X-ray to confirm position.

7. Technique—Removal:

a. Turn off IABP.

b. Aspirate air from balloon to ensure deflation.

c. Cut securing sutures and remove IABP catheter with a single swift pull.
d. Immediately place pressure over the insertion site with gauze pads in each hand. One hand is placed proximal to the entry site and one distal.
e. Release pressure from the distal hand to allow a little back bleeding from distal vessel in order to dislodge any clot present (Fig. 3.15).

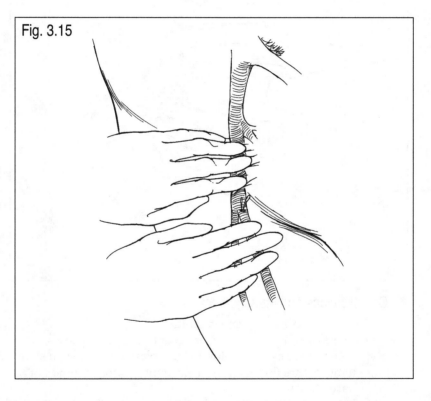

Fig. 3.15

f. Apply pressure with the distal hand and then release pressure from the proximal hand for 1–2 seconds allowing forward bleeding to dislodge clots (Fig. 3.16).
g. Hold manual pressure at both sites for a minimum of 30 minutes (Fig. 3.17).
h. The patient should remain supine with the legs extended for 6 hours.
i. Make frequent checks of the groin area for hematoma formation.
j. Monitor distal pulses regularly.

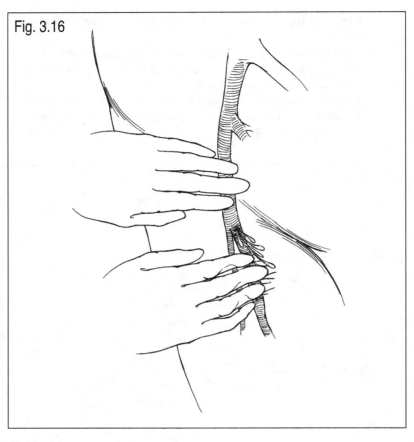

Fig. 3.16

8. Complications and Management:

a. Limb ischemia of lower extremities
- Manifested by decreased or absent peripheral pulses, a pale or blue skin discoloration, a relative decrease in skin temperature of the affected extremity, extremity pain or paresthesias.
- Document pre- and post-insertion pedal pulses. Assess the risk-benefit ratio of removing the IABP versus loss of limb.

b. Aortic dissection
- Caused by an intimal tear and flap made in the aorta during balloon insertion.
- Manifested by a poor augmentation tracing, failure of the balloon to unwrap, hypotension, or back pain.
- Immediately remove the IABP and initiate appropriate surgical treatment.

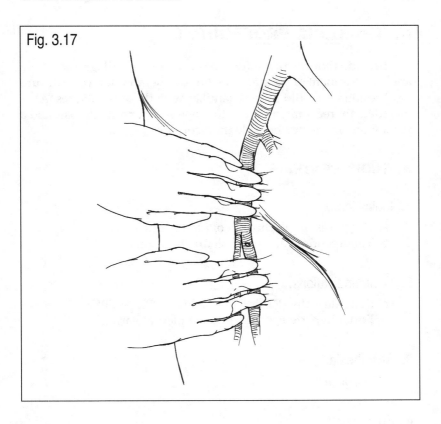

Fig. 3.17

c. Renal injury
   • Results either from thromboembolic events or secondary to occlusion of the orifice of the renal artery by the balloon.
   • Thrombectomy or proper repositioning of the balloon
d. Thromboembolism
   • May lead to limb or organ ischemia and may be prevented with anticoagulation.
   • Embolectomy is sometimes successful.
e. Bleeding
   • Usually occurs at the insertion site, particularly if the patient is anticoagulated or has a coagulopathy.
   • Often readily controlled with local pressure dressing.
f. Infection
   • Remove IABP.
   • Begin systemic antibiotics.

II. THORACIC PROCEDURES

Bedside thoracic procedures basically involve diagnosis and/or treatment of pleural effusions or pneumothoraces. All surgical residents should be very familiar with these techniques. Also included are recommendations for chemical pleural sclerosis and a section on emergency bedside thoracotomy.

A. THORACENTESIS

1. Indications:
a. Diagnosis of the etiology of pleural effusions
b. Therapeutic drainage of pleural effusions

2. Contraindications:
a. Coagulopathy (PT or PTT > 1.3 ratio, PLT < 50K)
b. Portal hypertension (producing pleural varices).

3. Anesthesia:
1% lidocaine

4. Equipment:
a. Sterile prep solution
b. Sterile gloves and towels
c. 22 and 25 gauge needles
d. 18 gauge insertion needle
e. 16 gauge single lumen central line and dilator
f. 0.035 "J" wire
g. Fine scissors
h. Nonvented IV tubing
i. Extension tubing
j. Three-way stopcock
k. 20 mL syringe
l. Vacuum bottles

5. Positioning:
Sitting erect on the edge of the bed resting with head and extended arms rested on a bedside table (Fig. 3.18)

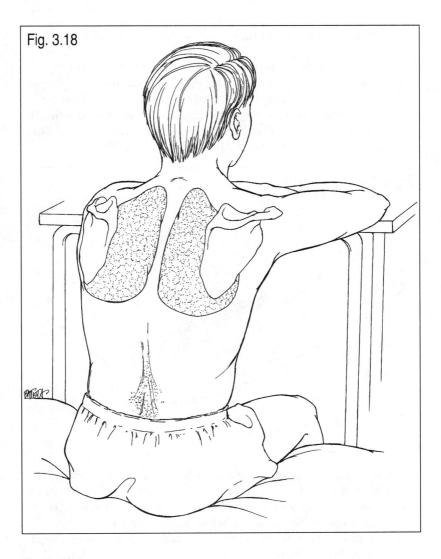

Fig. 3.18

6. Technique:

a. Percuss the hemithoraces and identify the bottom of the un-
   affected lung field and the meniscus of the affected lung
   field. Mark these landmarks on the patient's skin.

b. Prep and drape the patient's back.

c. Locate the posterior rib two interspaces below the top of the
   effusion, but not below the 8th intercostal space. Raise a skin
   wheal with a 25 gauge needle and 1% lidocaine at that inter-
   space just below the tip of the scapula. Alternatively, anes-

thetize a point two fingerbreaths below the tip of the scapula.

d. Using a 22 gauge needle, infiltrate the skin down to and *including the rib periosteum*. Carefully advance the needle *superiorly over the edge of the rib* while continuously infiltrating with lidocaine. Once over the rib, slowly advance the needle into the chest while aspirating the syringe until pleural fluid is encountered; withdraw the needle (Fig. 3.19).

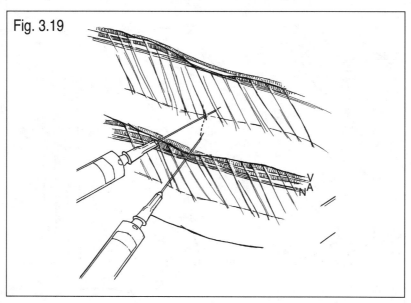

Fig. 3.19

e. Insert the 18 gauge insertion needle on a 20 mL syringe, with the *bevel directed inferiorly,* into the pleural cavity in the same manner slowly advancing the needle superiorly over the edge of the rib all the while aspirating. Once pleural fluid is encountered, remove the syringe and place a finger over the needle to prevent air from entering the pleural cavity.

f. Using the Seldinger technique, insert the wire through the needle into the chest and then carefully remove the needle leaving the wire (Fig. 3.20).

g. Introduce the dilator over the wire into the chest to dilate the subcutaneous tissues. Then remove the dilator.

h. With fine scissors, cut side holes in the distal one-third of the 16 gauge central line catheter encompassing no more than one-third of the catheter's diameter.

i. Insert the catheter into the chest over the wire and then re-

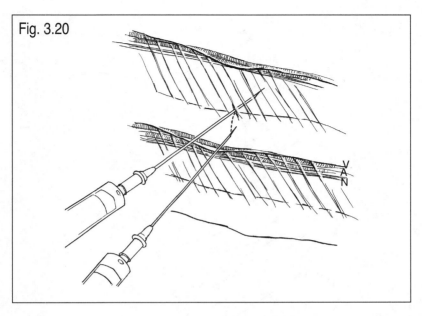

Fig. 3.20

move the wire. Keep a finger over the end of the catheter to
prevent air from entering the chest (Fig. 3.21).
j. Connect the extension tubing and vacuum apparatus (Fig.
3.22).
k. Open the stopcock and withdraw fluid. Position patient on
the side or back to improve flow.
l. Slowly withdraw catheter to remove any pockets of fluid located proximal to the tip until the catheter is pulled out of
the chest.
m. Obtain a chest X-ray to rule out pneumothorax and evaluate
remaining fluid.

7. Complications and Management:

a. Intercostal vessel damage
- By positioning the needle directly over the superior edge
of the rib, the risk is minimized.
- If a laceration occurs, monitor with serial chest X-rays. If the
hemothorax is significant, thoracostomy may be necessary.
b. Poor flow
- Rotate the patient in all directions to mobilize the thoracic
fluid.
- A bio-occlusive dressing may be placed over the insertion
site and the catheter allowed to stay in place for a period
of time.

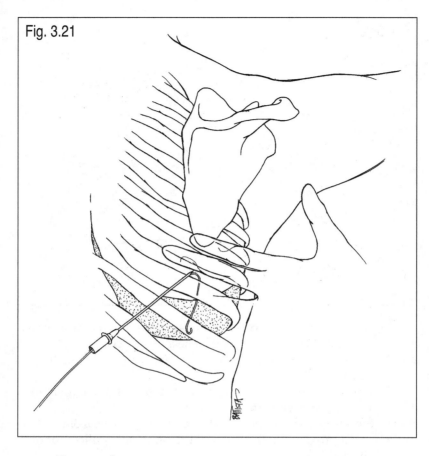

Fig. 3.21

c. Pneumothorax
- Keep air out of the system at all times.
- Monitor with serial chest X-rays. If the pneumothorax is significant (>10%), tube thoracostomy.

B. TUBE THORACOSTOMY

If there is *any question* of a *tension pneumothorax,* a 14 gauge or 16 gauge angio catheter should be *immediately* placed in the *2nd intercostal space in the midclavicular line* on the ipsilateral side before a chest X-ray and tube thoracostomy.

1. Indications:

a. Posterior chest tubes
- Hemothorax
- Significant pneumothorax (>15%)

Fig. 3.22

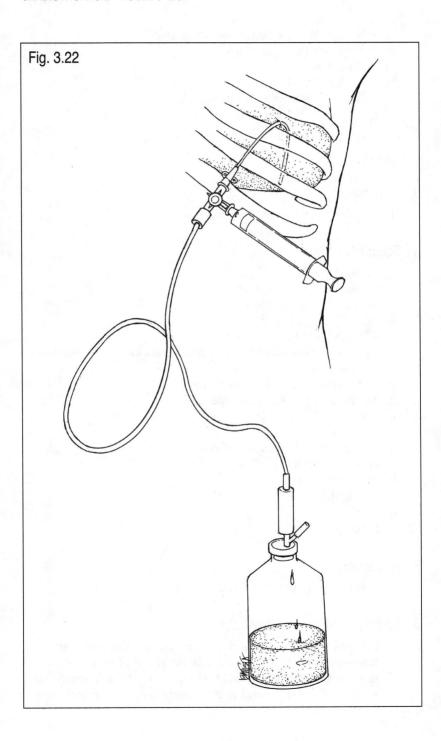

  - Symptomatic pneumothorax of any size
  - Persistent pleural effusion
  - Empyema
  b. Anterior chest tubes
    - Significant pneumothorax (>15%)

2. Contraindications:

None

3. Anesthesia:

1% lidocaine, IV sedation optional

4. Equipment:

  a. Sterile prep solution
  b. Sterile gloves and towels
  c. 3/4" 25 gauge needle
  d. 1/2" 22 gauge needle
  e. 60 mL syringe
  f. Chest tube #24–#28F for pneumothoraces and #34–#40F for fluid drainage
  g. 2–0 Vicryl sutures on cutting needles (2)
  h. #15 blade, long Kelly clamps (2)
  i. Long tonsillar clamp
  j. Heavy scissors
  k. A Pleur-evac filled with sterile water according to the accompanying insert
  l. Xeroform gauze
  m. Sterile dressing
  n. Cloth tape
  o. Benzoin solution

5. Positioning:

Supine with the ipsilateral arm raised above the head

6. Technique—Posterior Approach:

  a. Identify the *5th intercostal space* in the anterior axillary line—this is where the tube will enter the pleural space; however, the *incision is made at the level of the 6th intercostal space*. Generally, lateral to the nipple is approximately correct (Fig. 3.23).

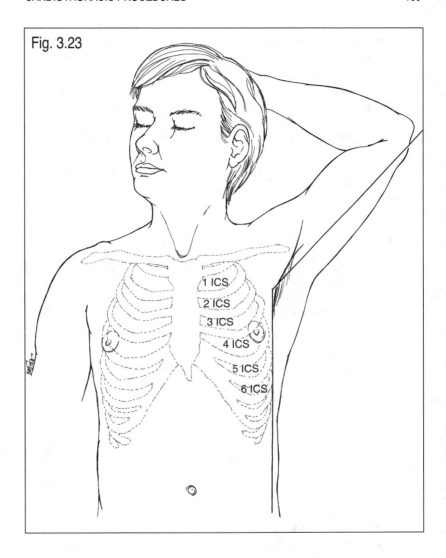

Fig. 3.23

1 ICS
2 ICS
3 ICS
4 ICS
5 ICS
6 ICS

b. Sterile prep and drape the hemithorax.

c. Using 1% lidocaine, raise a skin wheal with the 25 gauge needle and with the 22 gauge needle infiltrate the entire area. It is most important to infiltrate at the *level of the posterior periosteum and pleura.* This level can be located by drawing back slightly after entering the pleural space and obtaining air return with the 22 gauge finder needle.

d. Make a 1.5 cm horizontal incision down to subcutaneous fat.

e. Measure the chest tube on the outside of the patient's body and identify how far the tube should be advanced after placement. The tip of the tube should be at the *apex* of the lung, about 8–12 cm from the last hole in the chest tube in a 70 kg adult (Fig. 3.24).

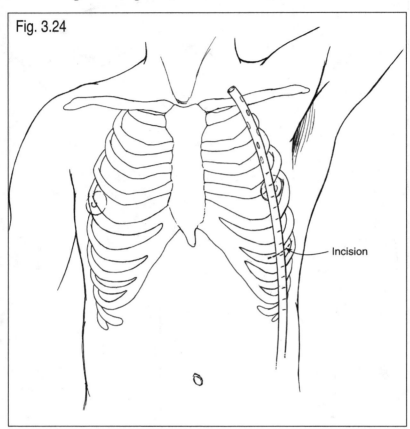

Fig. 3.24

Incision

f. With the tonsillar clamp, create a tract from the incision site superiorly, posteriorly, and immediately above the *superior edge* of the 6th rib to avoid injury to the neurovascular bundle (Fig. 3.25).
g. Upon entering the pleural space, a rush of air should be heard. Then, dilate the subcutaneous tract by spreading open the clamp.
h. Place a finger through the tract into the pleural space. Palpate the lung to confirm pleural cavity location and to assure that *no adhesions* are present. (The lung should expand and meet the palpating finger during inspiration.)
i. Place one Kelly clamp on the distal end of the chest tube.

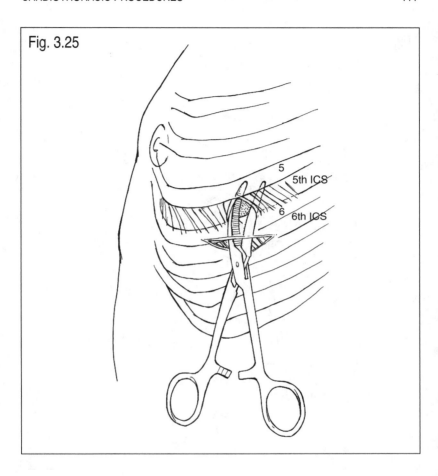

Fig. 3.25

j. Grasp the proximal end of the tube in the jaws of another
   Kelly and insert both through the subcutaneous tract into
   the pleural cavity. Direct the tube posteriorly toward the
   apex.
k. Open the jaws and remove the proximal Kelly while advancing the tube to the predetermined position (Fig. 3.26).
l. Attach the tube to the Pleur-evac and remove the distal
   Kelly. Secure the chest tube with two separate sutures. Place
   a horizontal mattress suture around chest tube and tape the
   untied ends of the suture around the tube to be used in closing the hole when the tube is removed. Place a piece of Xeroform gauze around the entrance site and a sterile dressing
   on top. Fasten securely with benzoin and cloth tape.
m. Confirm placement with a chest X-ray.

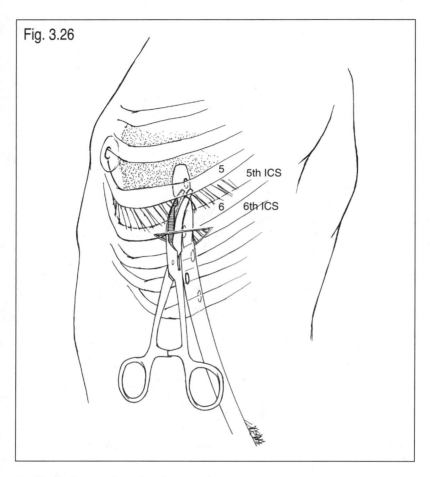

Fig. 3.26

7. Technique—Anterior Approach:

a. Obtain a #24 tube or smaller.
b. Identify the *2nd intercostal space* in the midclavicular line.
c. Sterile prep and drape the hemithorax.
d. Raise a skin wheal with the 25 gauge needle and with the 22 gauge needle infiltrate the entire area with 1% lidocaine. It is most important to infiltrate at the *level of the posterior periosteum and pleura*. This level can be located by drawing back slightly after entering the pleural space and obtaining air return with the 22 gauge finder needle.
e. Make a 1.5 cm horizontal incision down to subcutaneous fat.
f. Measure the chest tube on the outside of the patient's body and identify how far the tube should be advanced after placement.

g. With the tonsillar clamp, create a tract from the incision site superiorly, posteriorly, and immediately above the *superior edge* of the 3rd rib to avoid injury to the neurovascular bundle (Fig. 3.27).

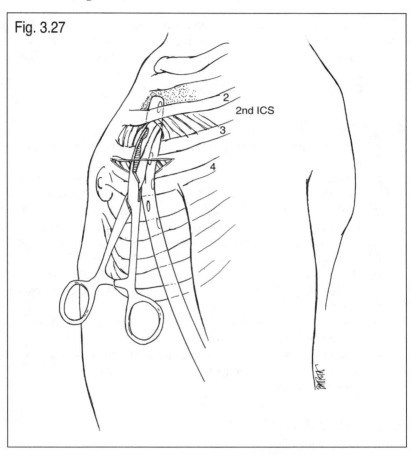

Fig. 3.27

h. Upon entering the pleural space, a rush of air should be heard. Then, dilate the subcutaneous tract by spreading open the clamp.

i. Place a finger through the tract into the pleural space. Palpate the lung to confirm pleural cavity location and to assure that *no adhesions* are present. (The lung should expand and meet the palpating finger during inspiration.)

k. Grasp the proximal end of the tube in the jaws of another Kelly and insert both through the subcutaneous tract into the pleural cavity. Direct the tube posteriorly toward the apex.

l. Open the jaws and remove the proximal Kelly while advancing the tube to the predetermined position.

m. Attach the tube to the Pleur-evac and remove the distal Kelly. Secure the chest tube with two separate sutures. Place a horizontal mattress suture around chest tube and tape the untied ends of the suture around the tube to be used in closing the hole when the tube is removed. Place a piece of Xeroform gauze around the entrance site and a sterile dressing on top. Fasten securely with benzoin and cloth tape.

n. Confirm placement with a chest X-ray.

8. Technique—Chest Tube Removal:

a. Cut the sutures anchoring the tube in position. Be careful not to cut the untied horizontal mattress suture.

b. Obtain Xeroform gauze and sterile gauze dressing to place over the insertion site. Place the dressing over the site.

c. While maintaining constant pressure seal on the skin with the gauze, promptly pull the chest tube out during exhalation. This prevents air from entering the pleural cavity and causing an iatrogenic pneumothorax.

d. Have an assistant maintain the pressure seal on the skin while you tie the horizontal mattress suture, thereby closing the skin.

e. Place a dressing on top of the site. The sutures can be removed in 1 week.

f. Obtain a chest X-ray to rule out an iatrogenic pneumothorax or a previously unappreciated air leak causing a pneumothorax.

9. Complications and Management:

a. Poor positioning
- The tube should be at the apex of the pleural cavity. It frequently gets trapped in the major fissure of the lung.
- Withdraw tube and re-insert.

b. Persistent pneumothorax
- Make sure all clamps are off the tubes and connection lines and that there is not an *obstruction* in the system.
- Check for an *air leak* in the system by clamping the tube at the chest wall. Air bubbling in the waterseal chamber indicates a leak. Change the Pleur-evac system.
- Repeat chest X-ray in 4 hours. If still present, higher suction up to −60 cm can be achieved with an Emerson

pump. If still no success then a second tube should be placed via the anterior approach.

c. Hemorrhage or lung injury
- Monitor chest tube output and obtain serial chest X-ray every 2 hours.
- Thoracotomy if hemodynamically unstable or if output is >300 mL/hr or 2L total

d. Cardiac dysrhythmias
- Withdraw chest tube 1–3 cm if adjacent to heart. If still persists, withdraw and re-insert via a separate skin site.
- Medical management if necessary

C. TROCAR CATHETER ("PIGSTICKER") TUBE THORACOSTOMY

If there is *any question* of a *tension pneumothorax,* a 14 gauge or 16 gauge angio catheter should be *immediately* placed in the *2nd intercostal space in the midclavicular line* on the ipsilateral side before a chest X-ray and tube thoracostomy.

1. Indications:

a. Small (<15%) pneumothorax when there is believed to be no or minimal air leak

2. Contraindications:

a. A standard chest tube should be placed rather than a trocar catheter in the following situations:
- Hemothorax
- Significant pneumothorax (>15%)
- Persistent pleural effusion
- Empyema

3. Anesthesia:

1% lidocaine, IV sedation optional

4. Equipment:

a. Sterile prep solution
b. Sterile gloves and towels
c. 3/4" 25 gauge needle
d. 1/2" 22 gauge needle
e. 60 mL syringe

   f. Argyle Trocar catheter 20F–24F

   g. 2–0 Vicryl sutures on cutting needles(2)

   h. #15 blade and scalpel handle

   i. Kelly clamp

   j. Heavy scissors

   k. A Pleur-evac filled with sterile water according to the insert

   l. Xeroform gauze

   m.Sterile dressing

   n. Cloth tape

   o. Benzoin solution

5. Positioning:

Supine with the ipsilateral arm raised above the head

6. Technique—Posterior Approach:

a. Identify the *5th intercostal space* in the anterior axillary line—this is where the tube will enter the pleural space; however, the *incision is made at the level of the 6th intercostal space.* Generally, lateral to the nipple is approximately correct (Fig. 3.28).

b. Sterile prep and drape the hemithorax.

c. Using 1% lidocaine, raise a skin wheal with the 25 gauge needle and with the 22 gauge needle infiltrate the entire area. It is most important to infiltrate at the *level of the posterior periosteum and pleura.* This level can be located by drawing back slightly after entering the pleural space and obtaining air return with the 22 gauge finder needle.

d. Make a 0.5 cm horizontal incision down to subcutaneous fat.

e. Measure the chest tube on the outside of the patient's body and identify how far the tube should be advanced after placement. The tip of the tube should be at the *apex* of the lung, about 8–12 cm from the last hole in the chest tube in a 70 kg adult.

f. Grasp the base of the trocar portion of trocar catheter in the palm of the right hand. This hand will supply the driving force of the insertion. The trocar should be fully advanced within the catheter (Fig. 3.29).

g. Grasp the tip of the trocar catheter with the left hand and insert the unit through the incision.

h. Using the left hand as a guide, apply gentle force with the right hand onto the trocar to tunnel the trocar catheter un-

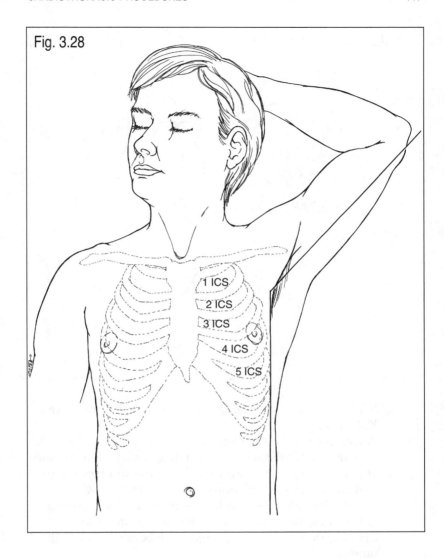

Fig. 3.28

1 ICS
2 ICS
3 ICS
4 ICS
5 ICS

der the skin over the *superior edge* of the 6th rib, avoiding injury to the neurovascular bundle (Fig. 3.30).

i. Upon entering the pleural space, a rush of air should be heard. Then, *gently* advance the entire unit not more than 2–3 cm into the pleural cavity aiming for the apex. Too much force or excessive advancement can result in lung injury.

j. Advance the *catheter only* over the trocar (hold the trocar stationary with the right hand) into the pleural space posteriorly toward the apex to the desired length (Fig. 3.31).

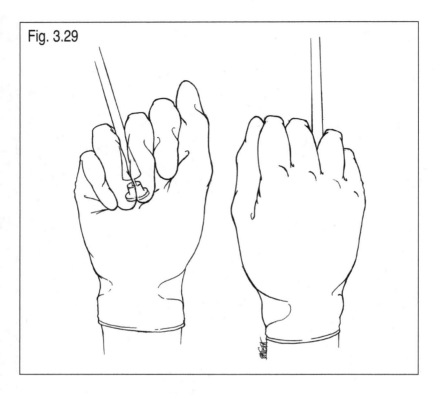

Fig. 3.29

k. Withdraw the trocar and clamp the end of the tube with a Kelly clamp.
l. Attach the tube to the Pleur-evac and remove the Kelly. Secure the chest tube with two separate sutures. Place a horizontal mattress suture around chest tube and tape the untied ends of the suture around the tube to be used in closing the hole when the tube is removed. Place a piece of Xeroform gauze around the entrance site and a sterile dressing on top. Fasten securely with benzoin and cloth tape.
m. Confirm placement with a chest X-ray.

7. Technique—Anterior Approach:

a. Identify the *2nd intercostal space* in the midclavicular line.
b. Sterile prep and drape the hemithorax.
c. Raise a skin wheal with the 25 gauge needle and with the 22 gauge needle infiltrate the entire area with 1% lidocaine. It is most important to infiltrate at the *level of the posterior periosteum and pleura*. This level can be located by drawing back

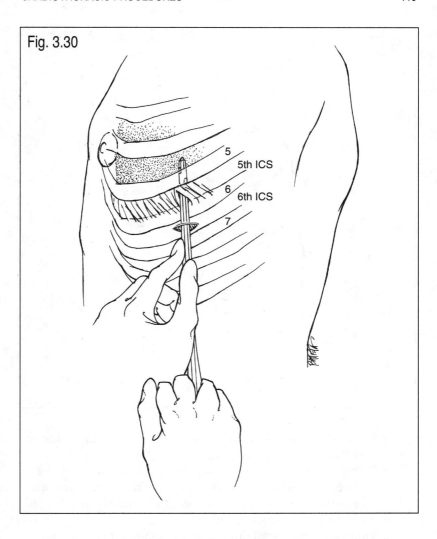

Fig. 3.30

slightly after entering the pleural space and obtaining air return with the 22 gauge finder needle.

d. Make a 0.5 cm horizontal incision down to subcutaneous fat.

e. Measure the chest tube on the outside of the patient's body and identify how far the tube should be advanced after placement.

f. Grasp the base of the trocar portion of trocar catheter in the palm of the right hand. This hand will supply the driving force of the insertion. The trocar should be fully advanced within the catheter (Fig. 3.32).

Fig. 3.31

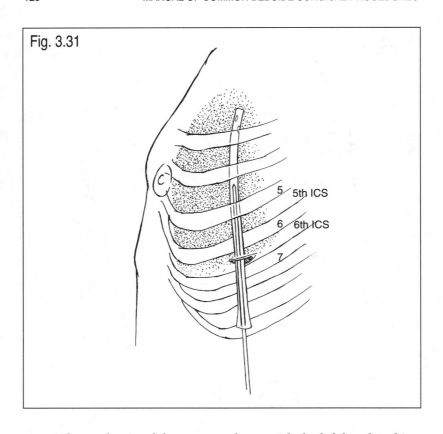

5 5th ICS

6 6th ICS

7

g. Grasp the tip of the trocar catheter with the left hand and insert the unit through the incision.

h. Using the left hand as a guide, apply gentle force with the right hand onto the trocar to tunnel the trocar catheter under the skin over the *superior edge* of the 3rd rib, avoiding injury to the neurovascular bundle.

i. Upon entering the pleural space, a rush of air should be heard. Then, *gently* advance the entire unit not more than 2–3 cm into the pleural cavity aiming for the apex. Too much force or excessive advancement can result in lung injury.

j. Advance the *catheter only* over the trocar (hold the trocar stationary with the right hand) into the pleural space posteriorly toward the apex to the desired length (Fig. 3.33).

k. Withdraw the trocar and clamp the end with a Kelly clamp.

l. Attach the tube to the Pleur-evac and remove the Kelly. Secure the chest tube with two separate sutures. Place a hori-

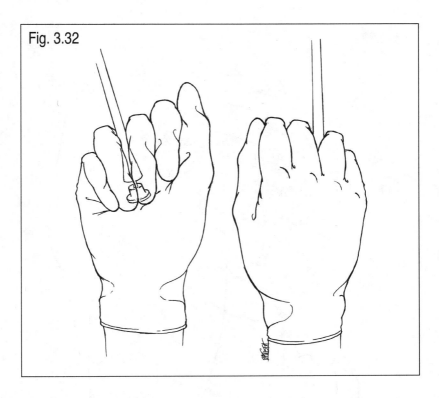

Fig. 3.32

zontal mattress suture around chest tube and tape the untied ends of the suture around the tube to be used in closing
the hole when the tube is removed. Place a piece of Xeroform gauze around the entrance site and a sterile dressing
on top. Fasten securely with benzoin and cloth tape.
m. Confirm placement with a chest X-ray.

8. Complications and Management:
a. Poor positioning
 - The tube should be at the apex of the pleural cavity. It frequently gets trapped in the major fissure of the lung.
 - If so, withdraw tube and re-insert.
b. Persistent pneumothorax
 - Make sure all clamps are off the tubes and connection
   lines, and that there is not an *obstruction* in the system.
 - Check for an *air leak* in the system by clamping the tube at
   the chest wall. Air bubbling in the waterseal chamber indicates a leak. Change the Pleur-evac system.

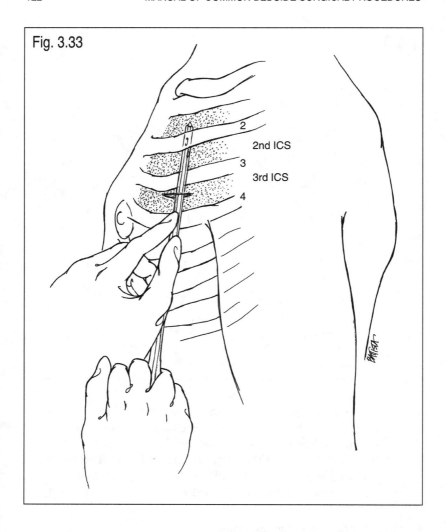

Fig. 3.33

- Repeat chest X-ray in 4 hours. If still present, higher suction up to −60 cm can be achieved with an Emerson pump. If still no success then a standard posterior tube thoracostomy should be performed.
  c. Hemorrhage or lung injury
    - Monitor chest tube output and obtain serial chest X-ray every 2 hours.
    - Thoracotomy if hemodynamically unstable or if output is >300 mL/hr or 2L total
  d. Cardiac dysrhythmias
    - Withdraw chest tube 1–3 cm if adjacent to heart. If still

persists withdraw and re-insert via a separate skin site.
- Medical management if necessary

D. CHEMICAL PLEURAL SCLEROSIS

1. Indications:
a. Persistent pneumothorax (persistent air leak with the lung expanded)
b. Recurrent malignant pleural effusions
c. Recurrent spontaneous pneumothoraces (relative)
d. Primary spontaneous pneumothorax (controversial)

2. Contraindications:
a. Allergies to tetracycline, doxycycline, or talc

3. Anesthesia:
1% lidocaine (50 mL)

4. Equipment:
a. Kelly clamp
b. Sterile prep solution
c. Gauze
d. Sterile normal saline
e. Doxycycline or talc
f. 60 mL syringes (2)

5. Positioning:
Supine initially. Patient must have a chest tube and Pleur-evac in place.

6. Technique—Doxycycline
a. Obtain doxycycline 500 mg in 50 mL normal saline and 40 mL 1% lidocaine in two separate 60 mL syringes.
b. Clamp the chest tube with a Kelly clamp near the entrance site at the skin.
c. Sterile prep the distal portion of the chest tube at the connection with the Pleur-evac tubing, and then disconnect the chest tube from the Pleur-evac.

   d. Attach the 60 mL syringe containing the lidocaine to the end of the chest tube.

   e. Remove the Kelly clamp, instill the lidocaine through the chest tube into the pleural cavity, and reclamp the chest tube.

   f. Rotate the patient from side to side every 2 minutes for 10–15 minutes to distribute the lidocaine for anesthesia.

   g. Fill the other 60 mL syringe with the doxycycline solution.

   h. Attach the doxycycline syringe to the chest tube, remove the Kelly clamp, and instill the solution into the pleural cavity. Clamp the chest tube.

   i. Repeat steps (g) and (h) until 300–400 mL of doxycycline have been administered.

   j. Rotate the patient to each of the following 4 positions every 30 minutes:
- Left lateral decubitus
- Right lateral decubitus
- Trendelenburg
- Reverse Trendelenburg

   k. After 4 hours, replace the chest tube back to Pleur-evac suction for at least the next 24 hours, until the lung has fully expanded and no air leak is present.

7. Technique—Talc

   a. Talc pleural sclerosis has been shown to result in a lower recurrence rate of spontaneous pneumothorax than doxycycline. Also, talc is generally less painful to the patient than doxycycline.

   b. Obtain talc 5 gm suspended in 250 mL normal saline and 40 mL 1% lidocaine in two separate 60 mL syringes.

   c. Clamp the chest tube with a Kelly clamp near the entrance site at the skin.

   d. Sterile prep the distal portion of the chest tube at the connection with the Pleur-evac tubing, and then disconnect the patient's chest tube from the Pleur-evac.

   e. Attach the 60 mL syringe containing the lidocaine to the end of the chest tube.

   f. Remove the Kelly clamp, instill the lidocaine through the chest tube into the pleural cavity, and reclamp the chest tube.

   g. Rotate the patient from side to side every 2 minutes for 10–15 minutes to distribute the lidocaine for anesthesia.

   h. Fill the other 60 mL syringe with the talc solution.

   i. Attach the talc syringe to the chest tube, remove the Kelly

clamp, and instill the solution into the pleural cavity. Clamp the chest tube.
j. Repeat steps (g) and (h) until all 250 mL of talc have been administered.
k. Rotate the patient to each of the following 4 positions every 30 minutes:
   • Left lateral decubitus
   • Right lateral decubitus
   • Trendelenburg
   • Reverse Trendelenburg
l. After 4 hours, replace the chest tube back to Pleur-evac suction for at least the next 24 hours, until the lung has fully expanded and no air leak is present.

E. EMERGENCY BEDSIDE THORACOTOMY

1. Indications:
a. Blunt or penetrating trauma in patients who have vital signs in the field and subsequent acute deterioration or cardiac arrest on arrival or during resuscitation
b. Cardiac arrest or profound hypotension secondary to tamponade (pericardiocentesis is not of practical value in acute circumstances).

2. Contraindications:
None

3. Anesthesia:
None

4. Equipment:
a. Sterile prep solution
b. Sterile gloves and towels
c. #10 blade and scalpel handle
d. Chest wall retractor
e. Mayo scissors
f. Metzenbaum scissors
g. Smooth forceps
h. Toothed forceps

    i. Aortic clamp

    j. Suction apparatus.

5. Positioning:

Supine

6. Technique:

    a. With a scalpel, make an incision at the level of the left 5th intercostal space in the midclavicular line.

    b. Carry the incision down to bone directly over the 5th rib and extend it from sternum to as far laterally as practical (Fig. 3.34).

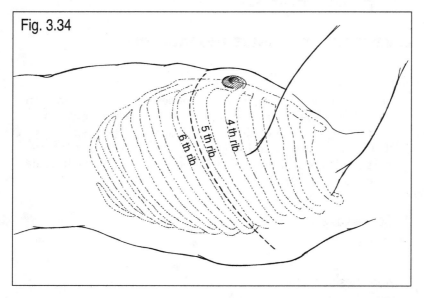

Fig. 3.34

    c. Insert partially opened Mayo scissors and run over the superior aspect of the 5th rib to open the thorax.

    d. Insert the chest wall retractor.

    e. Elevate the left lung out of the hemithorax to expose the descending thoracic aorta (Fig. 3.35).

    f. Bluntly dissect the mid-descending thoracic aorta circumferentially free from the posterior mediastinum and place an aortic clamp on it, being careful not to injure the esophagus anteriorly. A *nasogastric tube* (Chapter 4) can be placed to help distinguish the esophagus from the aorta on palpation. Drop the lung back into the hemithorax (Fig. 3.36).

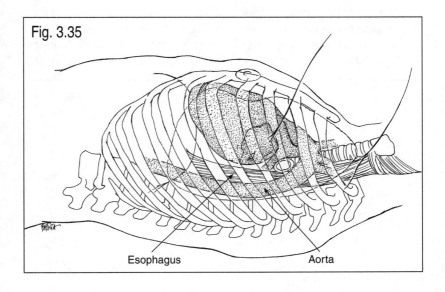

Fig. 3.35

Esophagus   Aorta

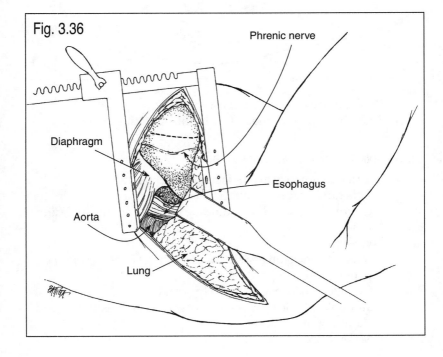

Fig. 3.36

Phrenic nerve

Diaphragm

Esophagus

Aorta

Lung

g. Open the pericardial sac in a longitudinal manner above the phrenic nerve from the diaphragm to the great vessels.

h. Manually evacuate any clot in the pericardium, and deliver the heart into the left hemithorax for examination (Fig. 3.37).

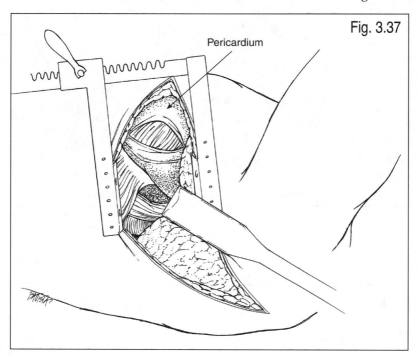

Fig. 3.37

Pericardium

i. Repair any cardiac wounds at this time.

j. Take the patient immediately to the operating room.

7. Complications and Management:

a. Internal mammary artery laceration (expected)
  • This rarely causes enough bleeding to be a problem in the emergency room, but should be repaired in the operating room.

b. Poor exposure
  • Make the incision as wide as is practical considering the patient's supine position
  • Get help. Have assistants help with lighting, instruments, and holding the lung out of the way during exposure and clamping of the aorta.
  • Make a large pericardiotomy.

c. Where to look for hemorrhage
- Penetrating trauma: (1) Follow the holes and do not forget that the lung could be a major source of bleeding. (2) If bleeding is from the pulmonary vessels, crossclamp the entire hilum.
- Blunt trauma: (1) Deceleration injuries—myocardial rupture at the insertion of the venae cavae (right atrium) and pulmonary veins (left atrium) or aortic tear at the ligamentum arteriosum. (2) Direct blow—right ventricular rupture at the origin of the pulmonary artery

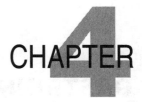

CHAPTER 4

GASTROINTESTINAL PROCEDURES

Authors: Peter Mattei, M.D. and Juan E. Sola, M.D.

GASTROINTESTINAL PROCEDURES

Disorders of the abdomen are, in many ways, the essence of true general surgery. The surgeon should have expertise in the anatomy of the abdomen and confidence in examination of the abdomen. By the same measure, gastrointestinal procedures should be an integral part of the armamentarium of the surgeon.

I. GASTROINTESTINAL TUBES

The purpose of gastrointestinal (GI) tubes is to evacuate the stomach (and occasionally more distal gastrointestinal tract) of gases and fluids for diagnostic and/or therapeutic purposes, or to deliver nutrients or medications. Modern GI tubes have a rich history; they are the product of many years' modifications in materials and design.

A. NASOGASTRIC TUBE

1. Indications:
   a. Acute gastric dilatation
   b. Gastric outlet obstruction
   c. Ileus
   d. Small bowel obstruction
   e. Upper gastrointestinal bleeding
   f. Enteral feeding

2. Contraindications:

a. Recent esophageal or gastric surgery
b. Absence of gag reflex

3. Anesthesia:

None

4. Equipment:

a. Levin or Salem sump tube
b. cup of ice
c. water soluble lubricant
d. catheter tip 60 mL syringe
e. cup of water with a straw
f. stethoscope

5. Positioning:

Sitting or supine

6. Technique:

a. Measure tube from mouth to earlobe and down to anterior abdomen so that last hole on tube is below xiphoid process. This marks the distance the tube should be inserted.
b. Place tip of tube in cup of ice to stiffen it.
c. Apply lubricant liberally to tube.
d. Ask patient to flex neck and gently insert tube into a patent naris (Fig. 4.1).
e. Advance tube into pharynx aiming posteriorly, asking the patient to swallow if possible.
f. Once the tube has been swallowed, confirm that the patient can speak clearly and breathe without difficulty and gently advance tube to estimated length. If the patient is able, instruct him or her to drink water through a straw; while the patient swallows, gently advance the tube.
g. Confirm correct placement into stomach by injecting approximately 20 mL of air with catheter tip syringe while auscultating epigastric area. Return of a large volume of fluid through tube also confirms placement into stomach.
h. Carefully tape tube to patient's nose ensuring that pressure is not applied by tube against naris. Tube should be kept well lubricated in order to prevent erosion at naris. With the

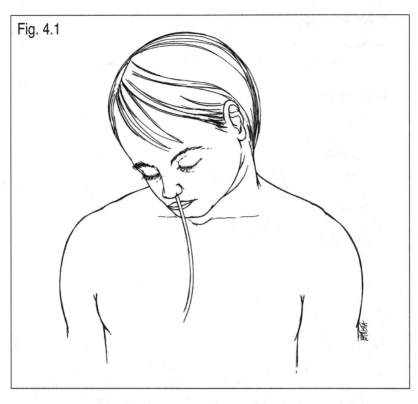

Fig. 4.1

use of tape and a safety pin, the tube can be secured to the patient's gown.

i. Irrigate tube with 15 mL of saline every 4 hours. Salem sump tubes will also require the injection of 15 mL of air through sump (blue) port every 4 hours in order to maintain proper functioning.

j. Constant low suction may be applied to Salem sump tubes, while Levin tubes should have only low intermittent suction.

k. Monitor gastric pH every 4–6 hours and correct with antacids for pH <4.5.

l. Monitor gastric residuals if tube is used for enteral feeding. Obtain a chest X-ray to confirm correct placement before using any tube for enteral feeding.

7. Complications and Management:

a. Pharyngeal discomfort
- Common due to the large caliber of these tubes.
- Throat lozenges or sips of water or ice may provide relief.

- Avoid using aerosolized anesthetic for the pharynx as this may inhibit the gag reflex, thereby eliminating the protective mechanism of the airway.
  b. Erosion of naris
    - Prevented by keeping tube well lubricated and ensuring that tube is taped so that pressure is not applied against naris. Tube should always be lower than the nose and never taped to the forehead of the patient.
    - Frequent checking of the tube position at the naris can help prevent this problem.
  c. Sinusitis
    - Occurs with long-term use of GI tubes.
    - Remove the tube and place in other naris.
    - Antibiotic therapy if needed.
  d. Nasotracheal intubation
    - Results in airway obstruction which is fairly easy to diagnose in the awake patient (cough, inability to speak).
    - Obtain a chest X-ray to confirm placement prior to use for enteral feeding.
  e. Gastritis
    - Usually manifests itself as mild, self-limited upper gastrointestinal bleeding.
    - Prophylaxis consists of maintaining gastric pH >4.5 with antacids via the tube, IV histamine$_2$ receptor blockers, and removal of tube as soon as possible.
  f. Epistaxis
    - Usually self-limited.
    - If persists, remove the tube and assess location of bleed.
    - Refer to Chapter 1 for treatment of anterior and posterior epistaxis.

B. OROGASTRIC TUBE

1. Indications:

The indications for orogastric (OG) tubes are generally the same as for NG tubes. However, because they are generally not tolerated well by the awake patient, they are used in intubated patients and newborns.
  a. Acute gastric dilatation
  b. Gastric outlet obstruction
  c. Ileus
  d. Small bowel obstruction

    e. Upper gastrointestinal bleeding
    f. Enteral feeding

2. Contraindications:
    a. Recent esophageal or gastric surgery

3. Anesthesia:
  None

4. Equipment:
    a. Levin or Salem sump tube
    b. water soluble lubricant
    c. catheter tip 60 mL syringe
    d. stethoscope

5. Positioning:
  Supine

6. Technique:
    a. Measure tube from mouth to earlobe and down to anterior abdomen so that last hole on tube is below xiphoid process. This marks the distance tube should be inserted.
    b. Apply lubricant liberally to tube.
    c. Because the patients in whom orogastric tubes are used are generally unable to cooperate, the tube should be placed into the mouth, directed posteriorly, until the tip begins to pass downward into the esophagus.
    d. Advance the tube slowly and steadily. If any resistance is encountered, stop and withdraw the tube completely. Repeat step c.
    e. If the tube advances easily, with little resistance, continue until the premeasured distance is reached. Resistance, gagging, fogging of the tube, or hypoxia suggests errant placement of the tube into the trachea.
    f. Confirm correct placement into stomach by injecting 20 mL of air with the catheter tip syringe while auscultating over the epigastric area. Correct placement is also confirmed by aspiration of a large volume of fluid.
    g. Irrigate tube with 15 mL of saline every 4 hours. Salem

sump tubes will require the injection of 15 mL of air through the sump (blue) port every 4 hours in order to maintain proper functioning.

h. Constant low suction may be applied to Salem sump tubes, while Levin tubes should have only low intermittent suction.

i. Monitor gastric residuals if tube is used for enteral feeding. Obtain a chest X-ray to confirm placement before using for enteral feeding.

7. Complications and management:

a. Pharyngeal discomfort and gagging is a problem with orogastric tubes when they are placed in awake and alert patients, and essentially eliminates their use in such patients.

b. Tracheal intubation
- Correct placement in the esophagus is usually evident by the ease of advancement of the tube. Any resistance suggests tracheal intubation or coiling within the posterior pharynx.
- Before initiating enteral feedings, the position of the oropharyngeal tube should be confirmed by chest X-ray.

c. Gastritis
- Usually manifests itself as mild, self-limited upper gastrointestinal bleeding.
- Prophylaxis consists of maintaining gastric pH >4.5 with antacids via the tube, IV histamine$_2$ receptor blockers, and removal of the tube as soon as possible.

C. NASODUODENAL TUBE

1. Indications:

a. Enteral feeding

2. Contraindications:

a. Recent esophageal or gastric surgery
b. Absence of gag reflex

3. Anesthesia:

None

4. Equipment:
   a. Tip-weighted, small-caliber tube
   b. Guide wire
   c. Water-soluble lubricant
   d. cup of water with a straw
   e. stethoscope
   f. Catheter tip syringe

5. Positioning:
   Sitting or supine

6. Technique:
   a. Measure tube from mouth to earlobe and down to anterior abdomen so that tip is 6 cm below xiphoid process.
   b. Most tips of duodenal tubes are self-lubricating when moistened with water. If not self-lubricating, apply water-soluble lubricant to the tip of the tube.
   c. Ask patient to flex neck and gently insert the tube containing the guide wire into a patent naris.
   d. Advance tube into pharynx aiming posteriorly, asking the patient to swallow if possible.
   e. Once the tube has been swallowed, confirm that the patient can speak clearly and breathe without difficulty and gently advance tube to estimated length. If the patient is able, instruct him or her to drink water through a straw and, while the patient swallows, gently advance the tube.
   f. Confirm correct placement into stomach by injecting approximately 20 mL of air with catheter tip syringe while auscultating the epigastric area.
   g. Remove the guide wire and ask the patient to lie in a right decubitus position for 1–2 hours. An abdominal radiograph at this point may confirm the presence of the tip in the duodenum or that the tube is coiled in the stomach and may need to be withdrawn for some distance. The tube should not be fixed to the nose.
   h. The patient should first lie in a supine position for 1–2 hours and then in a left decubitus position for 1–2 hours to facilitate passage of the tube through the C-loop of the duodenum.
   i. At this point, position of the tube should be confirmed by chest or abdominal X-ray. If the tube has not passed beyond the stomach by this time, placement of the tip may be neces-

sary through the pylorus by flexible upper endoscopy or under fluoroscopy.

7. Complications and Management:

   a. Epistaxis
     • Usually self-limited.
     • If persists, remove the tube and assess location of bleed.
     • Refer to Chapter 1 for treatment of anterior and posterior epistaxis.
   b. Intestinal perforation
     • Presents usually as free air on chest X-ray.
     • Caused by inserting guide wire back through lumen of tube while it is in place. *This should never be done.*
   c. Obstruction of lumen
     • Prevented by frequent flushing of tube with water or saline at regular intervals.
     • Clearing of obstruction should be attempted with saline or carbonated liquids using a 1 or 3 mL syringe.
     • The guide wire should *never be replaced* to clear an obstruction.

D. SMALL BOWEL TUBE

1. Indications:

   a. Early partial small bowel obstruction.

2. Contraindications:

   a. Uncooperative patient
   b. Indication for operative intervention (i.e., small bowel ischemia)

3. Anesthesia:

   None

4. Equipment:

   a. Long intestinal tube
   b. Water soluble lubricant
   c. Saline
   d. 5 mL syringe, 22 gauge needle

5. Positioning:

Sitting up initially, then variable position as described below.

6. Technique:

a. Using needle and syringe, inject 5 mL of saline into the balloon at the end of the tube (Fig. 4.2).

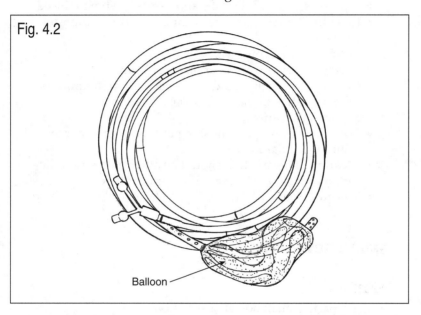

Fig. 4.2

Balloon

b. With the patient in an upright sitting position, roll up the balloon, apply a liberal amount of lubricant, and insert it into a patent naris.
c. Carefully manipulate the tube such that the balloon falls into the nasopharynx *without obstructing the airway.*
d. Instruct the patient to swallow the balloon as it is lowered slowly into the pharynx as though it were a bolus of food. Passage of the balloon in the patient who cannot swallow can be difficult. Often the balloon will advance along with the tube.
e. After it has been swallowed, confirm that the patient can speak clearly and breathe easily, then advance it slowly into the stomach by instructing the patient to continue swallowing.
f. Insert the tube to the point at which the "D" mark is at the nose, and have the patient lie in a right decubitus position for 1–2 hours. The tube should not be fixed to the nose. Low intermittent suction may be applied.

    g. Obtain an abdominal X-ray to confirm the presence of the tip in the duodenum or that the tube is coiled in the stomach and may need to be withdrawn for some distance.

    h. The patient should then be placed supine for 1–2 hours then next in a left decubitus position for 1–2 additional hours to facilitate passage of the tube through the C-loop of the duodenum.

    i. At this point, position of the tube should be confirmed again by abdominal X-ray. If the tube has not passed beyond the stomach by this time, placement of the tip through the pylorus may be necessary by flexible upper endoscopy or under fluoroscopy.

    j. Once the tube is in the duodenum, it can be advanced 2–3 cm every 15 minutes.

    k. Once the tube is no longer needed, removal should proceed slowly over *several hours in order to prevent intussusception* (withdraw tube 3–5 cm every 10–15 minutes).

7. Complications and Management:

    a. Airway obstruction
- The balloon may occlude the upper airway during initial placement.
- Withdraw the tube immediately.

    b. Epistaxis
- Usually self-limited.
- If it persists, remove the tube and assess location of bleed.
- Refer to Chapter 1 for treatment of anterior and posterior epistaxis.

    c. Intussusception of small intestine during removal
- Best avoided by withdrawing tube 3–5 cm every 10–15 minutes.

E. SENGSTAKEN-BLAKEMORE TUBE

The Sengstaken-Blakemore (SB) tube is an emergently placed tube that temporarily stops life-threatening hemorrhage from gastroesophageal varices. It is only a temporizing procedure before definitive operative or endoscopic therapy.

1. Indication:

    a. Exsanguinating hemorrhage from gastroesophageal varices

2. Contraindications:

None

3. Anesthesia:

None

4. Equipment:

a. Sengstaken-Blakemore (SB) tube
b. Catheter tip 60 mL syringe
c. Hemostat clamps (2)
d. Pressure manometer
e. Levine or Salem sump nasogastric tube
f. Water soluble lubricant
g. Scissors

5. Positioning:

Supine or lateral decubitus

6. Technique:

a. Because potentially lethal complications can occur with the use of the SB tube, patients should be in a monitored setting, such as the ICU, staffed by personnel experienced with the use of this device.
b. Control of the airway by endotracheal intubation is strongly advised to minimize the risk of aspiration.
c. Pass a large nasogastric tube (see section I.A) or orogastric tube (see section I.B) to empty the stomach of blood and then remove the tube.
d. Inflate both esophageal and gastric balloons with air to test for leaks.
e. Apply lubricant liberally to the tube.
f. Ask patient to flex neck and gently insert tube into a patent naris.
g. Advance tube into pharynx aiming posteriorly, asking the patient to swallow if possible.
h. Once the tube has been swallowed, confirm that the patient can speak clearly and breathe without difficulty and gently advance tube to approximately 45 cm.
i. Apply *low intermittent* suction to the gastric aspiration port. Return of blood should confirm placement in the stomach.

Otherwise inject 20 mL of air with the catheter tip syringe while auscultating epigastric area.

j. Slowly inject 100 mL of air into the gastric balloon and the clamp the balloon port to prevent air leakage. *Stop inflating the balloon immediately* if the patient complains of pain because this could indicate that the balloon is in the esophagus. If this is the case, deflate the gastric balloon, advance the tube an additional 10 cm, and repeat the injection of air.

k. With the gastric balloon inflated, slowly withdraw the tube until resistance is met at the gastroesophageal junction. Anchor the tube to the patient's nose under minimal tension with padding.

l. Obtain a chest X-ray to confirm correct gastric balloon position.

m. Add an additional 150 mL of air to the gastric balloon and reapply the clamp (Fig. 4.3).

n. Irrigate the gastric port with saline. If no further gastric bleeding is found, leave the esophageal balloon deflated.

o. If bleeding persists, connect the esophageal balloon port to the pressure manometer and inflate the esophageal balloon to 25–45 mm Hg.

p. Transiently deflate the esophageal balloon every 4 hours to check for further bleeding (by aspirating through the gastric port) and to prevent ischemic necrosis of the esophageal mucosa.

q. Apply low intermittent suction to both the gastric and esophageal aspiration tubes.

r. After 24 hours without evidence of bleeding (stable vital signs and hemoglobin), deflate the esophageal and gastric balloons.

s. The SB tube can be removed after an additional 24 hours without evidence of bleeding.

7. Complications and Management:
    a. Esophageal perforation
        • Can result from intraesophageal inflation of the gastric balloon.
        • Deflate the gastric balloon and remove the SB tube.
        • Emergent surgical consult for operative therapy.
    b. Aspiration
        • Prevented by endotracheal intubation
        • Supportive therapy (oxygen, chest PT)
        • Appropriate antibiotics

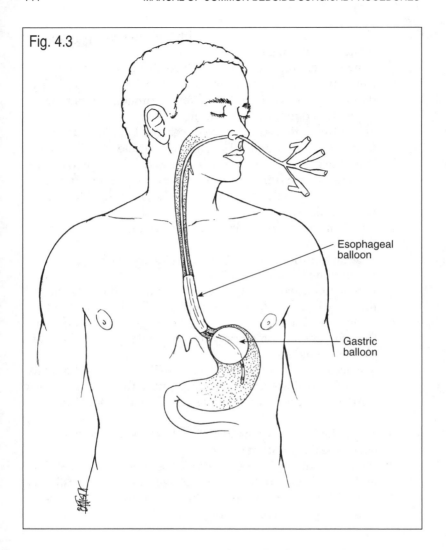

Fig. 4.3

Esophageal balloon

Gastric balloon

    c. Rebleeding following SB tube removal
- Reinsert SB tube
- Endoscopy or definitive surgery

II. LOWER GASTROINTESTINAL PROCEDURES

    The anus and rectum are readily examined at the bedside using a number of straightforward techniques. Likewise, many lesions of the anorectal region are easily dealt with in the awake patient without the need for general anesthesia or operating room equipment. Although often considered "minor procedures," the direct benefit to the patient is often immense.

A. ANOSCOPY

1. Indications:
   a. Anal lesions (fistulas, tumors, etc.)
   b. Rectal bleeding
   c. Rectal pain
   d. Banding or injection of hemorrhoids

2. Contraindications:
   a. Massive lower GI bleeding
   b. Anal stricture
   c. Acute perirectal abscess
   d. Acutely thrombosed hemorrhoid

3. Anesthesia:
   None

4. Equipment:
   a. Clear polyethylene anoscope
   b. Water soluble lubricant
   c. Directed light source or head-light.

5. Positioning:
   Lateral decubitus position or lithotomy position

6. Technique:
   a. Examine anus by gently spreading anoderm and performing digital rectal examination.
   b. Insert the anoscope slowly, using liberal amounts of lubricant and with the obturator in place, until the flange at the base rests on perianal skin.
   c. Remove the obturator and, while withdrawing the anoscope, examine the anal mucosa in a systematic manner.

d. Replace the obturator prior to removal of the anoscope.
e. Repeat the procedure as needed to ensure full inspection of the anal canal.

7. Complications and Management:

a. Fissure
  • Anal or perianal tears can occur and usually respond to conservative measures, such as stool softeners and Sitz baths.
b. Bleeding
  • Unusual but may occur, especially in the setting of large internal hemorrhoids; it is usually self-limited.

B. RIGID SIGMOIDOSCOPY

1. Indications:

a. Rectal bleeding
b. Lower abdominal and pelvic trauma
c. Extraction of foreign bodies
d. Stool cultures
e. Evaluation and biopsy of ileal pouch

2. Contraindications:

a. Massive lower GI bleeding
b. Anal stricture
c. Acute perirectal abscess
d. Acutely thrombosed hemorrhoids

3. Anesthesia:

None

4. Equipment:

a. Rigid sigmoidoscope and obturator
b. Light source
c. Suction apparatus
d. Insufflating bulb
e. Water soluble lubricant
f. Long cotton-tipped swabs
g. Biopsy forceps, if planning biopsy

5. Positioning:

Lateral decubitus, lithotomy, or prone jackknife

6. Technique:
   a. Administer tap water or saline enema before procedure to empty distal colon of feces.
   b. Perform a digital rectal examination to assess for masses.
   c. Assemble sigmoidoscope by placing the obturator through the scope. Check light source and suction. Lubricate the scope thoroughly with water soluble lubricant.
   d. Gently insert the sigmoidoscope through the anus to 5 cm, remove the obturator, and attach the light source.
   e. Judiciously insufflate air in order to visualize the lumen, using the *minimum* amount of air necessary to see.
   f. Advance the sigmoidoscope as a unit slowly to visualize the rectum. *Avoid* using the anus as a levering point. Air will leak during the procedure and intermittent insufflation will be necessary.
   g. The lumen of the sigmoid will be posterior toward the sacrum and then gently curving to the patient's left. To minimize the risk of perforation, advance the sigmoidoscope only when the lumen is clearly visualized.
   h. If stool is obstructing the view, use the cotton-tipped swabs to clear the lumen.
   i. Advance the sigmoidoscope under direct vision as far as tolerated by the patient (usually 20–25 cm) (Fig. 4.4).
   j. To biopsy a mass or polyp, advance the scope until part of the mass is within the barrel of the scope. Insert the biopsy forceps into the barrel and grasp a specimen of tissue. If needed, silver nitrate sticks can be used to achieve hemostasis.
   k. Closely and systematically inspect the mucosa while withdrawing the instrument slowly.

7. Complications and Management:
   a. Bleeding
      • Usually self-limited, but may follow biopsy.
      • Rarely will require treatment, but if bleeding is hemodynamically significant, then resuscitate and consider endoscopic treatment.
   b. Perforation
      • Manifested by abdominal pain, distention, and loss of hepatic dullness to percussion.

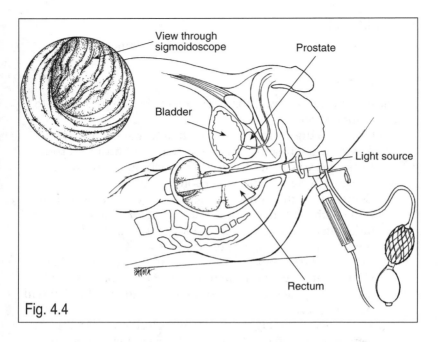

View through
sigmoidoscope

Prostate

Bladder

Light source

Rectum

Fig. 4.4

- Obtain upright chest X-ray; free air under the diaphragm
  confirms the diagnosis.
- NPO, IVF, IV antibiotics, operative management.

C. EXCISION OF THROMBOSED EXTERNAL HEMORRHOID

1. Indications:

    a. Thrombosed external hemorrhoid causing extreme pain

2. Contraindications:

    a. Coagulopathy (PT or PTT >1.3X ratio)
    b. Thrombocytopenia (PLT < 50K)
    c. Non-thrombosed prolapsed hemorrhoids

3. Anesthesia:

    1% lidocaine

4. Equipment:

    a. Scalpel handle and #15 blade
    b. Sterile prep solution

c. 25 gauge needle and syringe
d. Forceps
e. Small clamps

5. Positioning:

Lateral decubitus or lithotomy

6. Technique:

a. Attempt to sterile prep and drape the anal area and canal with sterile prep solution.
b. Identify the thrombosed external hemorrhoid. By definition, it lies exterior to the dentate line, and it is firm and tender (Fig. 4.5).

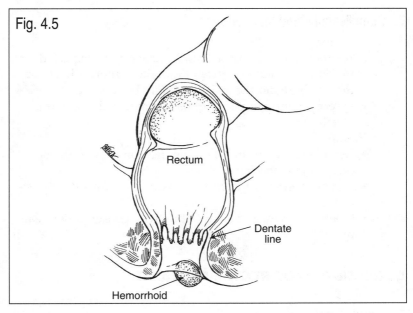

Fig. 4.5

Rectum

Dentate line

Hemorrhoid

c. Perform a field block of the hemorrhoid by infiltrating the surrounding skin and soft tissues with lidocaine using a 25 gauge needle.
d. Using a scalpel, make an elliptical incision over the thrombosed hemorrhoid (Fig. 4.6).
e. Using the forceps to hold one side of the incision, enucleate the clot within the hemorrhoid with the aid of a clamp. Apply a Vaseline gauze or xeroform dressing.
f. The patient should be instructed to do Sitz baths three times a day and after each bowel movement.

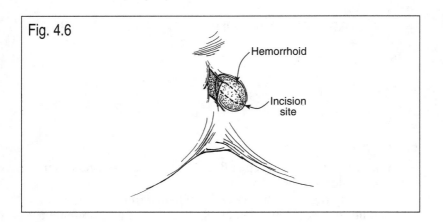

Fig. 4.6

Hemorrhoid

Incision
site

7. Complications and Management:

a. Bleeding
- A small amount of dark bloody ooze is to be expected. Bright red bleeding indicates that the hemorrhoid is not thrombosed and the incision should be stopped.
- Direct pressure or packing may be required to control bleeding.

b. Fissure
- Usually results from extending incision beyond the hemorrhoid into anoderm.
- Treat conservatively with Sitz baths and Anusol suppositories.
- Operative management if failure with conservative treatment.

D. REDUCTION OF RECTAL PROLAPSE

1. Indications:

a. Prolapse of rectum (full-thickness)
b. Mucosal prolapse of rectum (mucosa only)

2. Contraindications:

a. Infarction or gangrene of prolapsed segment
b. Severe tenderness of prolapsed segment
c. Extreme edema of prolapsed segment

3. Anesthesia:

None

4. Equipment:

a. Gloves
b. Water soluble lubricant

5. Positioning:

Decubitus or dorsal lithotomy

6. Technique:

a. Don gloves and apply a liberal amount of water soluble lubricant to the prolapsed segment.
b. The concept is to apply steady, circumferential pressure on the prolapsed segment (to decrease edema) while simultaneously trying to reduce it. This is done by placing as many fingers of both hands, oriented parallel to its longitudinal axis, around the segment and compressing it from all sides.
c. Apply pressure firmly and steadily, with more pressure applied at the tip than at the base.
d. Progress is typically slow and almost imperceptible. Be patient and squeeze for 1 to several minutes at a time, using plenty of lubricant.
e. To prevent recurrence, the patient should be placed on stool softeners and should be instructed in the technique of manual self-reduction of prolapsed hemorrhoids, which may occur at each bowel movement.

7. Complications and Management:

a. Unsuccessful reduction
  • May result in infarction of prolapsed segment
  • Requires surgical management with excision of prolapsed portion

III. ABDOMINAL PROCEDURES

These procedures are used to access the peritoneal cavity or to sample its contents. They are very useful techniques that can provide diagnostic information or therapeutic benefit without the need for a major operative procedure.

A. PARACENTESIS

1. Indications:

Removal of intra-abdominal fluid for:
a. Diagnostic studies
  - Ascites
  - Spontaneous bacterial peritonitis
b. Therapeutic purposes
  - Relief of respiratory compromise
  - Relief of pain and abdominal discomfort

2. Contraindications:

a. Coagulopathy (PT or PTT > 1.3)
b. Thrombocytopenia (plt < 50 000)
c. Bowel obstruction
d. Pregnancy
e. Infected skin or soft tissue at entry site

3. Anesthesia:

1% lidocaine

4. Equipment:

a. Sterile preparation solution
b. Sterile towels
c. Sterile gloves
d. 5 mL syringes, 20 mL syringes, 25 gauge and 22 gauge needles
e. 3-way stopcock, IV tubing
f. IV catheter (diagnostic: 20 gauge, therapeutic: 18 gauge), or long 16 gauge catheter with 0.035 cm "J" wire
g. 500–1000 mL vacuum bottles and IV drip set (for therapeutic paracentesis)

5. Positioning:

Supine
a. Preferred site of entry
  - Either lower quadrant (anterior iliac spine)
  - Lateral to the rectus muscle
  - At the level of or just below the umbilicus

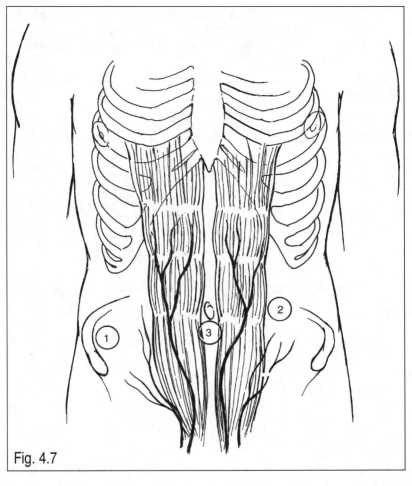

Fig. 4.7

    b. The entry site should not be the site of a prior incision and
      should be free of gross contamination and infection.
    c. The entry sites are percussed to confirm the presence of fluid
      and the absence of underlying bowel.

6. Technique—Diagnostic Sampling:
    a. Prepare site with sterile preparation solution and drape with
      sterile towels.
    b. Use 25 gauge needle to anesthetize skin and 22 gauge needle
      to anesthetize abdominal wall to peritoneum.
    c. Introduce IV catheter into the abdominal cavity, aspirating
      as you advance. The needle should traverse the abdominal
      wall at an oblique angle.

   d. When free flow of fluid occurs, the catheter should be advanced over the needle and the needle removed.

   e. Draw 20–30 mL of fluid into a sterile syringe for diagnostic studies and culture (Fig. 4.8).

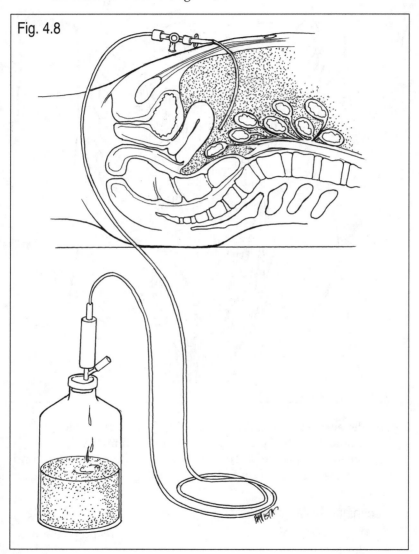

Fig. 4.8

   f. If less than an adequate volume is withdrawn, the catheter should be removed and replaced, possibly at another entry site.

7. Technique—Therapeutic Drainage:

a. Prepare site with sterile preparation solution and drape with sterile towels.

b. Use 25 gauge needle to anesthetize skin and 22 gauge needle to anesthetize abdominal wall to peritoneum.

c. Introduce IV catheter into the abdominal cavity, aspirating as you advance. The needle should traverse the abdominal wall at an oblique angle.

d. When free flow of fluid occurs, the catheter should be advanced over the needle and the needle removed. Alternatively, a long CVP-type catheter with extra side holes may placed over a guide wire using the Seldinger technique: After insertion of the needle and fluid is freely aspirated, a J-tip guide wire is placed through the needle, into the peritoneal space. The needle is removed, leaving the wire in place. A stiff plastic dilator is used to dilate the tract by placing it over the wire and into the abdomen. An 11-blade scalpel can be used to make a tiny nick at the entry site as well. The dilator is removed and the catheter is placed over the wire and into the abdomen and the wire is removed.

e. Draw 20–30 mL of fluid into a sterile syringe for diagnostic studies and culture. For therapeutic fluid removal, an IV drip set may be used with evacuated bottles or gravity drainage to remove a large volume of fluid.

f. Should the catheter become occluded, careful manipulation of the catheter to re-establish flow may be undertaken. Alternatively, asking the patient to turn on his or her side and again onto his or her back may also help re-establish flow. However, the needle or guide-wire should *not* be reintroduced because of the risk of bowel injury. If less than an adequate volume is withdrawn, the catheter should be removed and replaced, possibly at another entry site.

7. Complications and Management:

a. Hypotension:

- Can occur during or after procedure due to rapid mobilization of fluid from intravascular space or due to vasovagal response.
- Intravenous hydration can prevent and correct the hypotension in most cases.

- Removal of more than one liter of fluid is more likely to result in hypotension. This can be prevented by giving intravenous 5% albumin as replacement (e.g., 250 mL per liter of fluid removed).
  b. Bowel perforation
  - Rarely recognized at time of procedure
  - Can lead to infected ascites, peritonitis, and sepsis.
  c. Hemorrhage
  - Rare but can be caused by injury to mesentery or injury to inferior epigastric vessels.
  - Usually self-limited. Avoided by entering abdomen lateral to rectus.
  - For unstable hemodynamic bleeding, laparotomy.
  d. Persistent ascites leak
  - Usually will seal in <2 weeks. Can result in peritonitis.
  - Skin entry site may be sutured with figure 8 stitch to minimize leak.
  e. Bladder perforation
  - Avoided by inserting Foley catheter prior to procedure.
  - May require a period of bladder catheterization until sealed.
  - Obtain Urology consult.

B. DIAGNOSTIC PERITONEAL LAVAGE

1. Indications:
   a. Blunt abdominal injury, in the adult patient associated with:
      - Equivocal or unreliable abdominal exam (e.g., following head trauma or intoxication)
      - Suspicion for organ injury
      - Unexplained hypotension or blood loss
   b. short-term peritoneal dialysis

2. Contraindications:
   a. Indication for laparotomy
   b. Pregnancy
   c. Cirrhosis
   d. Morbid obesity
   e. Prior abdominal surgery

3. Anesthesia:
   1% lidocaine *with* epinephrine.

4. Equipment:

  a. Sterile preparation solution
  b. Sterile towels, sterile gloves, gown, mask, cap
  c. Syringes: 5 mL, 10 mL, 20 mL
  d. 25 gauge needle
  e. Peritoneal dialysis catheter
  f. IV tubing
  g. 1000 mL bag of normal saline or Ringer's lactate
  h. Scalpel handle and #10 and #11 (or #15) blades
  i. Surgical instruments: tissue forceps, hemostats, Allis clamps, retractors, suture

5. Positioning:

  Supine. The stomach should be decompressed by a *nasogastric* or an *orogastric* tube. The bladder should be drained by a *Foley catheter.*

6. Technique:

  a. Prepare the entire abdomen with sterile preparation solution and drape with sterile towels.
  b. With a 25 gauge needle and 1% lidocaine with epinephrine, anesthetize a site in the lower midline approximately one-third the distance from the umbilicus to the symphysis pubis (Fig. 4.9).
  c. Make a small incision down to the linea alba with a #10 blade. (The linea alba is midline in position and recognized by its decussating fibers and absence of muscle beneath it.)
  d. Incise the fascia in the midline for a length of approximately 1 cm, grasping the edges of the fascia with hemostats or Allis clamps (Fig. 4.10).
  e. Introduce the dialysis catheter into the peritoneal cavity at an oblique angle aiming towards the cul-de-sac and advance it carefully into the pelvis.
  f. Aspirate from the catheter with a syringe. Gross blood (5 mL or more) or gross enteric contents are indications for immediate laparotomy.
  g. If no gross blood or enteric contents are aspirated, instill 10 mL/kg of warmed saline or Ringer's lactate, up to 1000 mL, via the intravenous tubing. Appearance of fluid in chest tube drainage or Foley catheter drainage is also an indication for laparotomy.

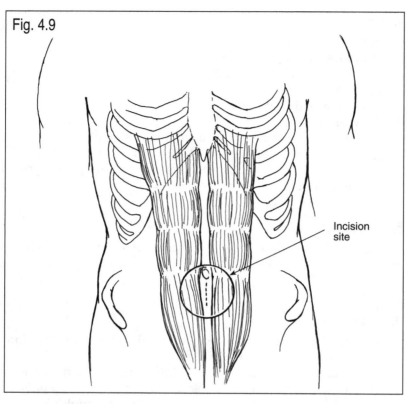

Fig. 4.9

Incision
site

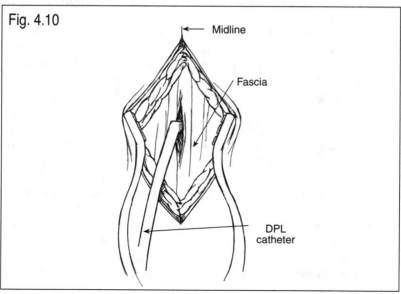

Fig. 4.10

Midline

Fascia

DPL
catheter

h. After waiting 5–10 minutes, allow the fluid to drain by gravity back into its original bag.

i. Send a sample of the fluid in the bag for cell count and amylase. Positive findings include a red blood cell count of >100,000/mm^3, a white blood cell count >500/mm^3, or amylase >175. *Note:* Criteria for positive lavage findings may vary among individual trauma surgeons and according to the mechanism of injury.

j. At the conclusion of the procedure, the catheter is removed and the fascia and skin are closed carefully using standard techniques (interrupted #1 Prolene, Vicryl, or PDS for fascia).

7. Complications and Management:

   a. Bladder injury
      - Preventable by inserting Foley catheter prior to procedure.
      - Treated by Foley catheter drainage for a period of several days.
   b. Injury to bowel or other abdominal organ
      - May require laparotomy for repair
      - Treated with NPO, IV hydration, IV antibiotics, laparotomy.
   c. Hemorrhage
      - Rarely life-threatening but may lead to false positive results, especially if source is skin or subcutaneous tissue.
      - treated with NPO, IV hydration, laparotomy if it persists.
   d. Peritonitis
      - May be due to poor aseptic technique or bowel perforation.
   e. Wound infection
      - A potential late complication. Incidence may be diminished by a dose of broad-spectrum IV antibiotics prior to procedure.

C. TENCKHOFF CATHETER INSERTION

1. Indications:

   Short-term or chronic ambulatory peritoneal dialysis.

2. Contraindications:

   a. Obliterated peritoneal space (prior surgery, infection, carcinomatosis)

  b. Ruptured diaphragm
  c. Respiratory insufficiency
  d. Presence of a large ventral or umbilical hernia

3. Anesthesia:

  1% lidocaine

4. Equipment:

  a. Sterile preparation solution
  b. Sterile towels and gloves
  c. Scalpel handle and #10 blade
  d. Tissue forceps
  e. Self-retaining retractor
  f. Double cuff peritoneal dialysis catheter
  g. 000 absorbable suture on a taper point curved needle
  h. 00 nylon suture on a curved cutting needle
  i. 25 gauge and 22 gauge needle
  j. 10 mL syringe

5. Positioning:

Supine. The stomach should be decompressed by a *nasogastric* or an *orogastric* tube. The bladder should be drained by a *Foley catheter*.

6. Technique:

  a. Prepare the entire abdomen with sterile preparation solution and drape with sterile towels.
  b. With a 25 gauge needle and lidocaine, anesthetize a site lateral to the midline (over the rectus abdominis) approximately one-third the distance from the umbilicus to the symphysis pubis.
  c. Make a longitudinal incision approximately 5 cm in length down to the level of fascia.
  d. Anesthetize a tract for the creation of a subcutaneous tunnel, to a point 8–12 cm lateral to the incision and make a small stab incision at this point (Fig. 4.11).
  e. Tunnel the dialysis catheter such that the proximal cuff lies in a subcutaneous location and the distal cuff lies in the first incision (Fig. 4.12).
  f. Make an incision in the fascia and retract the rectus laterally, exposing the posterior fascia.

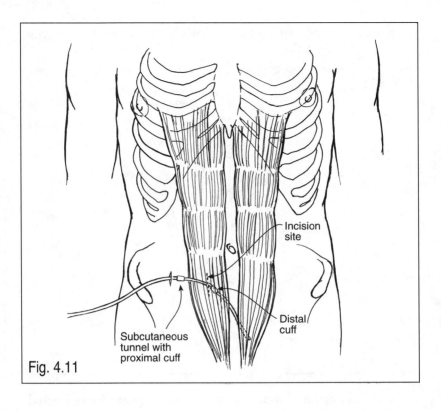

Fig. 4.11

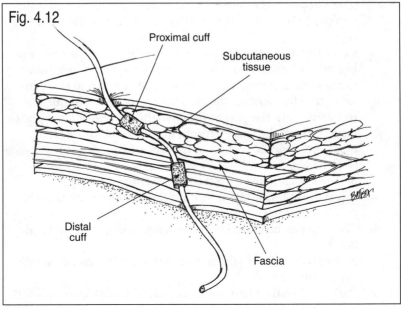

Fig. 4.12

g. Place a purse string of 000 absorbable suture in the posterior fascia (Fig. 4.13).

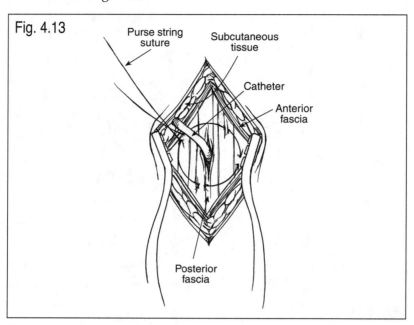

Fig. 4.13

Purse string suture

Subcutaneous tissue

Catheter

Anterior fascia

Posterior fascia

h. Under direct vision, carefully incise the posterior fascia and peritoneum in the center of the purse string suture. Locally explore to be certain that adhesions or viscera are not in the way.

i. Carefully insert the catheter into the peritoneal cavity, aiming inferior and posteriorly (towards the right lower quadrant), such that the distal cuff lies just anterior to the peritoneum. The catheter should feed easily and without resistance into the pelvis. Remove the obturator (stiff plastic insert). Flush the catheter with heparinized saline (100 units/mL) and be certain of the lack of significant resistance (Fig. 4.14).

j. Secure the catheter with the purse string suture.

k. Close the anterior fascia around the catheter such that the cuff lies within the muscle.

l. The skin can be closed in the usual fashion, preferably in layers.

m. Secure the catheter where it exits the smaller incision with skin sutures.

n. Peritoneal dialysis can begin the same day as long as small volumes (1 liter) are used.

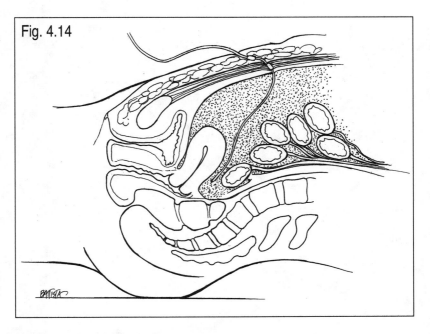

Fig. 4.14

7. Complications and Management:

a. Injury to intra-abdominal viscus
- May occur in the setting of extensive adhesions or previous surgery.

b. Peritonitis
- An ever-present risk that requires careful technique and surveillance.
- May occasionally require removal of catheter.

c. Catheter dysfunction
- Can be caused by ingrowth of tissue or adhesions to the catheter and usually requires catheter removal.
- Omentum is less likely to occlude the catheter if it is placed correctly deep in the pelvis.

CHAPTER 5

NEUROSURGICAL PROCEDURES

Author: Prakash Sampath, M.D.

NEUROSURGICAL PROCEDURES

Neurological surgery is a relatively new discipline that encompasses the surgical and medical management of diseases of the central nervous system (the brain, spinal cord, and their coverings) as well as diseases of the peripheral nervous system. In recent years, advancements in microsurgical techniques and neuroanesthesia have vastly broadened the scope of neurosurgical practice and have resulted in marked improvement in patient morbidity and outcome.

Neurosurgery is ostensibly a hospital-based specialty involving operations under general anesthesia, but there are several bedside procedures that are essential in patient diagnosis, management, and therapy. In this chapter, five common procedures are presented that may be encountered by any physician.

A. LUMBAR PUNCTURE

1. Indications:

    a. CSF analysis and sampling
    b. Drainage of cerebrospinal fluid (CSF)
    c. Measurement of opening pressure
    d. Intrathecal administration of contrast or drugs

2. Contraindications:

    a. Noncommunicating hydrocephalus
    b. Known or suspected intracranial mass (tumor, abscess, hematoma)

c. Coagulopathy or platelets <50K
d. Infection in the region of puncture
e. Complete spinal block (relative)
f. Children with tethered cord
g. Papilledema

3. Anesthesia:

1% lidocaine

4. Equipment:

a. Sterile prep solution
b. Sterile gloves and towels
c. 22 gauge and 25 gauge needles
d. 22 gauge, 20 gauge, or 18 gauge spinal needle with stylet
e. CSF collection vials
f. manometer with stopcock

5. Positioning:

a. If CSF opening pressure is required, the patient must be in the supine position with the knees to the chest and the head flexed.
b. The sitting position may be desirable in obese patients or where large volumes of CSF are to be collected.

6. Technique:

a. Sterile prep and drape entire region of lower back.
b. Identify the intercristal line, which connects the superior borders of the iliac crest, and palpate in the midline for the spinous processes (usually L4). The procedure can be attempted in L3–4, L4–5, and L5–S1 spaces (Figs. 5.1 and 5.2).
c. Inject superficially 1 mL 1% lidocaine one fingerbreadth below the spinous process of L4 (L4–5 space). Then, aiming slightly rostrally, inject 3 mL 1% lidocaine in the deep lumbodorsal fascia.
d. Puncture the skin using the spinal needle with the stylet over the anesthetized skin. The bevel of the needle should be anterior (Fig. 5.3).
e. Advance the needle deeper, aiming rostrally about 15° and taking care to maintain a midline trajectory (Fig. 5.4). The needle will encounter slight resistance, then a "pop" will be

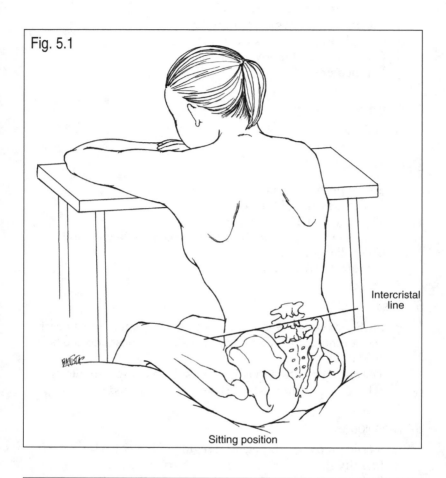

Fig. 5.1

Intercristal line

Sitting position

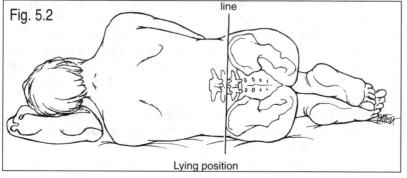

Fig. 5.2

line

Lying position

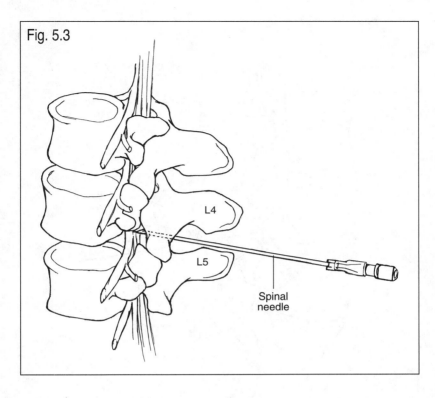

Fig. 5.3

L4

L5

Spinal
needle

felt representing penetration through the ligamentum
flavum into the thecal sac. (The stylet should *always* be used
with needle to prevent introduction of epidermoid cells or
subcutaneous tissue into thecal sac.)

f. If bone is encountered, it is more often due to *deviation from
the midline* as opposed to failure to aim in the correct rostral-
caudal direction. If this occurs, pull back needle 1–2 cm and
re-aim trajectory.

g. Once needle appears to be in thecal sac, remove stylet and
observe for CSF. If blood appears, allow blood to drain and
observe for clearance since this may simply represent a traumatic tap. If blood does not clear or no CSF is observed, replace stylet, withdraw needle, and re-attempt (Fig. 5.5).

h. If CSF flow is established, place stopcock on end of needle
with manometer. Ask patient to slowly straighten his or her
legs. Adjust stopcock to allow CSF to flow up manometer
and measure pressure in cm H_2O. (Patient's body must be
straight and as relaxed as possible to obtain accurate opening pressure.)

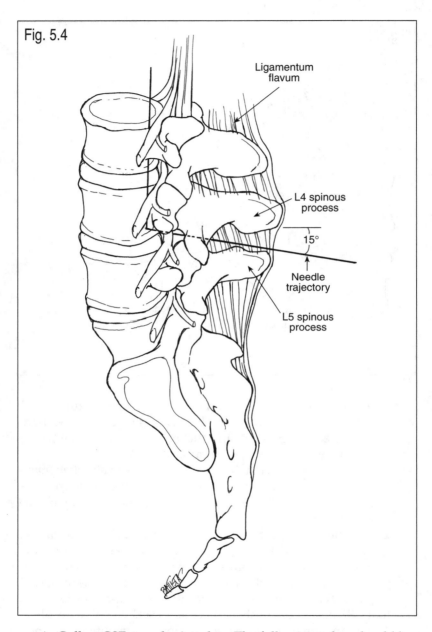

Fig. 5.4

Ligamentum flavum

L4 spinous process

15°

Needle trajectory

L5 spinous process

i. Collect CSF samples in tubes. The following tubes should be sent for analysis on every lumbar puncture performed:
- Cell count
- Protein and glucose
- Culture and sensitivity
- Cell count (to compare with tube 1)

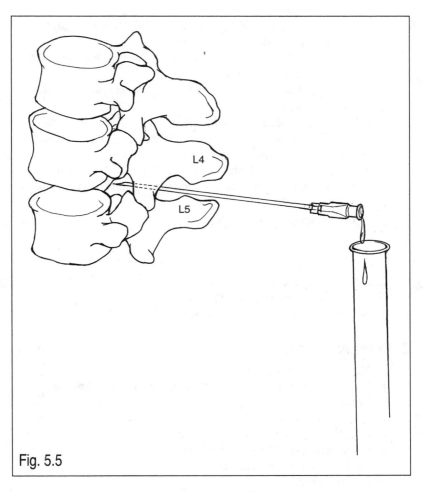

Fig. 5.5

j. Replace stylet and withdraw needle.
k. Place sterile gauze over puncture site. Changes in mental status, vital signs, and pupil size and reactivity must be carefully monitored.

7. Complications and Management:

a. Tonsillar herniation
   - Can manifest as dilating unilateral pupil, change in mental status, Cushing's triad (hypertension, bradycardia, decreased respiratory rate).
   - Immediately remove needle and raise the head of bed.
   - Administer diuretics (e.g., Lasix, mannitol) as needed.
   - Protect airway; hyperventilate as needed.
   - Emergent neurosurgical consult

    b. Nerve root injury (sudden pain radiating down the leg)
- Withdraw needle immediately.
- If pain persists start Decadron 4 mg every 6 hours for 24 hours. Taper off over 4 days.
- Consider EMG if pain persists for a few days.

    c. Spinal headache
- Keep the patient supine as tolerated.
- Usually resolves within hours but can persist for days.

    d. Aortic/arterial puncture
- Withdraw needle immediately and keep the patient supine for 4–6 hours while monitoring hemodynamics.

B. LUMBAR DRAIN PLACEMENT

1. Indications:
    a. CSF fistula or CSF leak
    b. Intrathecal pressure monitoring
    c. Normal pressure hydrocephalus (NPH)

2. Contraindications:
    a. Noncommunicating hydrocephalus
    b. Known or suspected intracranial mass (tumor, abscess, hematoma)
    c. Coagulopathy or platelets <50K
    d. Infection in the region of puncture
    e. Complete spinal block (relative)
    f. Children with tethered cord
    g. Papilledema

3. Anesthesia:
    1% lidocaine

4. Equipment:
    a. Sterile prep solution
    b. Sterile gloves and towels
    c. 14 gauge Touhy needle
    d. IV pressure tubing
    e. Lumbar drain
    f. CSF collection bag (e.g., bile bag)
    g. Ruler

5. Positioning:

The patient must be in the supine position with the knees to the chest and the head flexed.

6. Technique:

a. Sterile prep and drape entire region of lower back.
b. Identify the intercristal line, which connects the superior borders of the iliac crest, and palpate in the midline for the spinous processes (usually L4). The procedure can be attempted in *L3–4, L4–5,* and *L5–S1* spaces (Fig. 5.6).

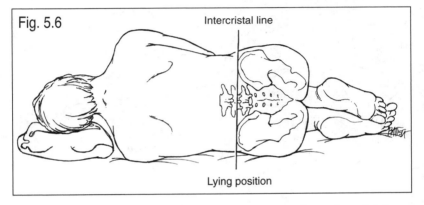

Fig. 5.6

Intercristal line

Lying position

c. Inject superficially 1 mL 1% lidocaine one fingerbreadth below the spinous process of L4 (L4–5 space). Then, aiming slightly rostrally, inject 3 mL 1% lidocaine in the deep lumbodorsal fascia.
d. Puncture the skin using the Touhy needle with the stylet over the anesthetized skin. The bevel of the needle should be anterior.
e. Advance the needle deeper, aiming rostrally about 15° and taking care to maintain a midline trajectory. The needle will encounter slight resistance, then a "pop" will be felt representing penetration through the ligamentum flavum into the thecal sac. (The stylet should *always* be used with needle to prevent introduction of epidermoid cells or subcutaneous tissue into thecal sac.)
f. If bone is encountered, it is more often due to *deviation from the midline* as opposed to failure to aim in the correct rostral-caudal direction. If this occurs, pull back needle 1–2 cm and re-aim trajectory.
g. Once needle appears to be in thecal sac, remove stylet and

observe for CSF. If blood appears, allow blood to drain and observe for clearance since this may simply represent a traumatic tap. If blood does not clear or no CSF is observed, replace stylet, withdraw needle, and re-attempt (Fig. 5.7).

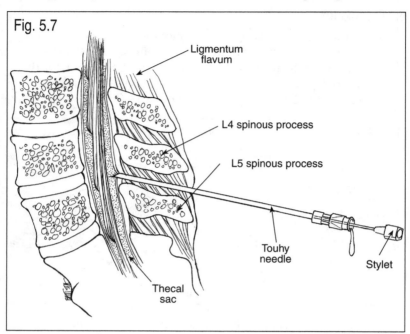

Fig. 5.7

h. If CSF flow is established, slowly withdraw stylet and feed 10 cm of the lumbar drain through the Touhy needle. The drain should now be in the thecal space (Fig. 5.8).
i. Slowly withdraw the Touhy needle and remove it over the lumbar drain, taking care to ensure the drain does not move.
j. Check to make sure the lumbar drain still drains CSF.
k. Place the connector to the free end of the drain and connect to the IV pressure tubing (Fig. 5.9).
l. Secure the drain to the patient's back with sterile dressing.
m. Lay the patient supine and set the desired drainage pressure using a ruler. The collection bag is placed at a given height above the lower back . (e.g., the standard is a "pop-off" of 10 cm. To achieve this, the bag should be placed 10 cm above the lower back).
n. If the pop-off is set too low and excessive CSF is drained, the patient may develop complications ranging from bad headaches to lethargy and even coma. Immediately *clamp off drain* if any symptoms of over-drainage develop.

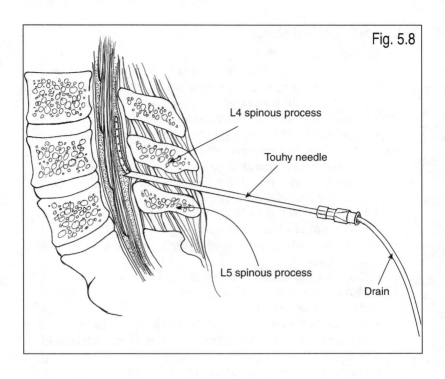

Fig. 5.8

L4 spinous process

Touhy needle

L5 spinous process

Drain

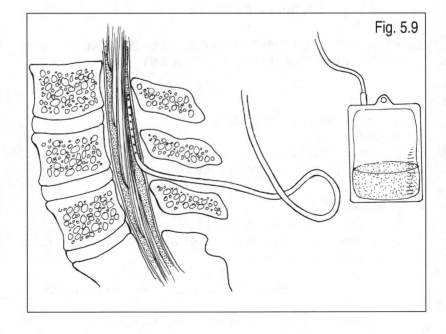

Fig. 5.9

7. Complications and Management:
   a. Tonsillar herniation
      - Can manifest as dilating unilateral pupil, change in mental status, Cushing's triad (hypertension, bradycardia, decreased respiratory rate).
      - Immediately remove needle and raise the head of bed.
      - Administer diuretics (e.g., Lasix, mannitol) as needed.
      - Protect airway; hyperventilate as needed.
      - Emergent neurosurgical consult
   b. Nerve root injury (sudden pain radiating down the leg)
      - Withdraw needle immediately.
      - If pain persists, start Decadron 4 mg every 6 hours for 24 hours. Taper off over 4 days.
      - Consider EMG if pain persists for a few days.
   c. Spinal headache
      - Keep the patient supine as tolerated.
      - Usually resolves within hours but can persist for days.
   d. Aortic/arterial puncture
      - Withdraw needle immediately and keep the patient supine for 4–6 hours while monitoring hemodynamics.
   e. Meningitis
      - Obtain CSF cultures, culture the drain, and promptly remove the drain.
      - Start CSF-penetrating antibiotics.

C. VENTRICULOSTOMY/INTRACRANIAL PRESSURE (ICP) MONITOR (BOLT) PLACEMENT

1. Indications:
   a. Direct measurement of ICP
   b. Hydrocephalus
   c. Drainage of CSF (with ventriculostomy)
   d. Drainage of blood in subarachnoid hemorrhage (SAH)

2. Contraindications:
   a. Posterior fossa lesions (relative)
   b. Patients with midline shift (Ventricular catheter placement may cause further brain shifts.)
   c. Coagulopathy or platelets <50k
   d. Vascular malformation or other mass lesion in the catheter path
   e. Aneurysmal subarachnoid hemorrhage (Draining CSF in-

creases the transmural pressure across an aneurysm and increases the risk of rupture.)

3. Anesthesia:

1% lidocaine, short acting IV sedation, and nondepolarizing paralytics if patient moving

4. Equipment:
a. Sterile prep solution
b. Sterile gloves and towels
c. 22 gauge and 25 gauge needles
d. 22 gauge spinal needle with stylet
e. Razors (2)
f. Bone wax
g. Sterile saline solution
h. Scalpel
i. 3–0 nylon suture
j. Needle driver
k. Scissors
l. Hand-held cranial twist drill
m. Standard ventricular catheter or Richmond bolt and/or intraparenchymal ICP monitoring device (e.g., Camino)
n. Sterile dressing

5. Positioning:

The patient should be supine with the head of the bed raised 20–25°. The head should be in the neutral position (Fig. 5.10).

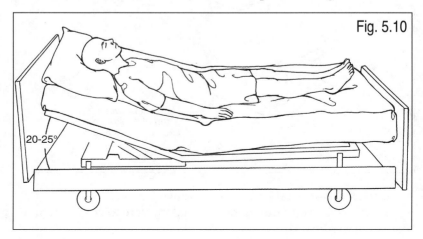

Fig. 5.10

20-25°

6. Technique:

   a. Shave the entire right side of the head and the left frontal portion.

   b. The right *Kocher's point* is the most commonly used site. This utilizes the nondominant hemisphere, lies anterior to the motor homunculus, and avoids injury to the superior sagittal sinus. To find Kocher's point, follow a perpendicular line up midway between the external auditory meatus and lateral canthus until you reach the midpupillary line on the right side. Alternatively, if the coronal suture is palpable, mark the intersection 2 cm anterior to the coronal suture and 4 cm lateral to midline (Fig. 5.11).

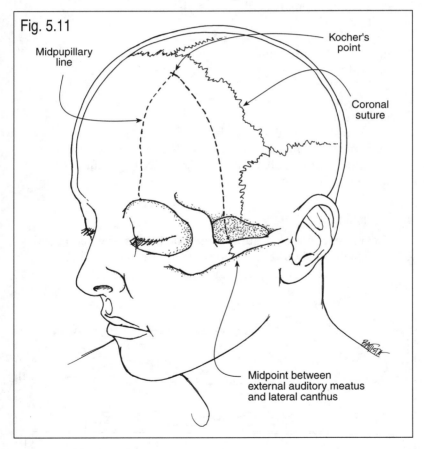

Fig. 5.11

Midpupillary line

Kocher's point

Coronal suture

Midpoint between external auditory meatus and lateral canthus

   c. Five minute sterile prep of the shaved areas.

   d. Drape the right frontal portion, taking care to clearly define the midline.

e. Make a 2 cm parasagittal incision over Kocher's point down to bone using the scalpel to scrape away and elevate the pericranium.

f. Use the twist drill to carefully make a hole in the skull, *taking care not to plunge into the brain* (Fig. 5.12).

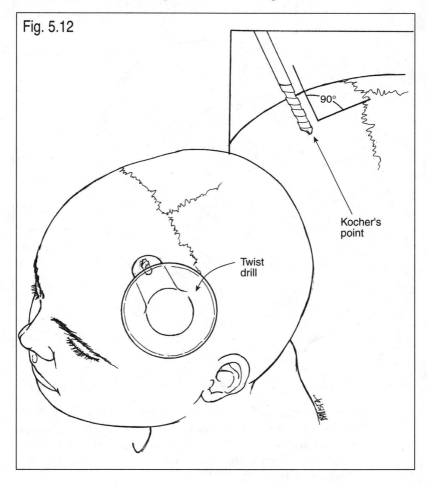

Fig. 5.12

90°

Kocher's point

Twist drill

g. Irrigate away the bone chips with saline solution and use bone wax to stop bone bleeding.

h. Puncture the underlying dura with the spinal needle and widen the dural incision a few millimeters (Fig. 5.13).

i. Insert ventricular catheter (IVC) with stylet *perpendicular* to brain surface to depth of 5–7 cm (Fig. 5.14).

j. Withdraw the stylet to ensure CSF flow. If *no CSF flow* is established, carefully replace stylet and advance catheter fur-

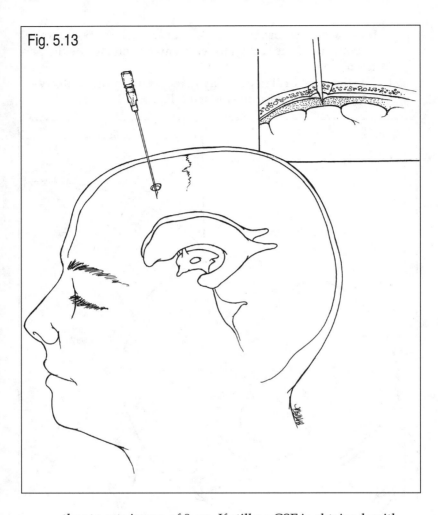

Fig. 5.13

ther to maximum of 9 cm. If still no CSF is obtained, withdraw catheter from brain and reassess trajectory. Studying a
CAT scan is often helpful in this regard. Usually aiming the
catheter slightly more medial is a safe and effective way to
establish CSF flow (Fig. 5.15).

k. If unsuccessful in obtaining CSF after three attempts, place a
subarachnoid bolt or intraparenchymal monitor instead.
   - For the *Richmond bolt*, screw in until the tip is flush with
     the inner table of the skull (Fig. 5.16).
   - For the *Camino* or other intraparenchymal monitoring de-
     vice, screw in stabilizing bolt and insert device 1.5–2 cm
     through the burr hole into the brain parenchyma.

l. Using a needle driver, tunnel IVC beneath the scalp to exit

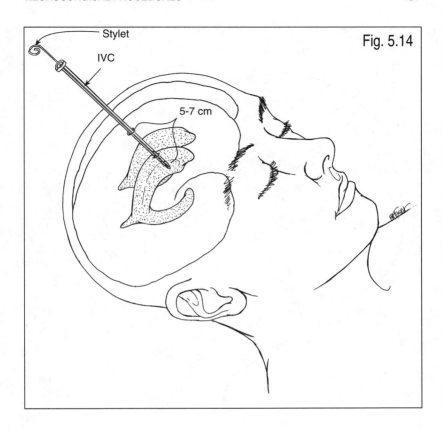

Fig. 5.14

Stylet

IVC

5-7 cm

through separate skin incision 2–3 cm posterior-lateral to Kocher's point. Confirm CSF flow after tunneling.
m. Connect the IVC or ICP monitor to the pressure transducer and/or drainage level. Set a fixed "pop-off" level for drainage using the ear as reference (e.g., place the bag 10 cm above the ear if that is the desired "pop-off").
n. Suture all incisions and secure IVC drain to scalp.
o. Use sterile dressing over entire frontal portion of scalp.

7. Complications and Management:
   a. Bleeding
      • If there is any change in neurologic exam, seizure, or un-expected blood seen after placement of IVC, an immediate head CT should be obtained.
      • Most IVC hemorrhages resolve spontaneously and require supportive care. Occasionally, the CT may reveal an aberrantly placed IVC that needs removal.

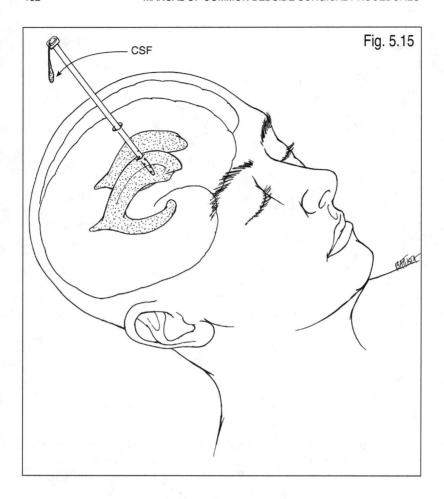

Fig. 5.15

CSF

- In very rare circumstances, operative evacuation of hematoma is indicated.
b. Infection
   - The reported risk of infection varies from 0 to 27%. CSF surveillance cultures should be taken daily.
   - Aggressive antibiotics
   - All IVCs and ICP monitors should be removed after 1 week and replaced if still needed.
c. Tonsillar herniation
   - Can manifest as dilating unilateral pupil, change in mental status, Cushing's triad (hypertension, bradycardia, decreased respiratory rate).
   - Immediately clamp off IVC.

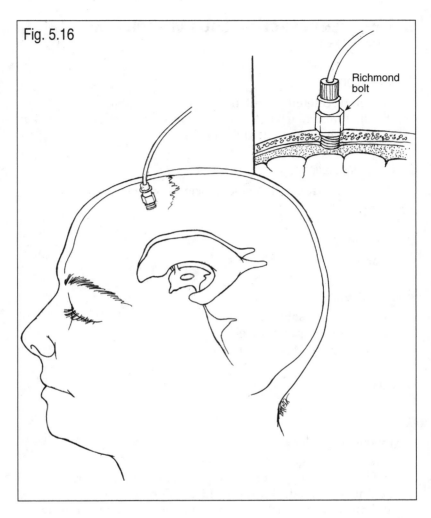

Fig. 5.16

Richmond bolt

- Intubate and hyperventilation.
- Mannitol (0.5–1 g/kg) and other diuretics
- Emergent neurosurgery consult
d. Aneurysm rupture
  - If bright red blood is suddenly seen draining from IVC, emergently place another IVC in other ventricle or perform emergent percutaneous ventricular puncture to maintain ventricular access.
  - Keep pop-off pressures high enough to minimize CSF drainage (usually in the 15–20 mm Hg range).
  - Emergent head CT and/or angiogram
  - Emergent neurosurgery consult

D. EMERGENT PERCUTANEOUS VENTRICULAR PUNCTURE

1. Indications:
   a. Life-threatening herniation from hydrocephalus
   b. Life-threatening ventriculo-peritoneal (V-P) shunt malfunction
   c. Massive subarachnoid hemorrhage

2. Contraindications:

   Only to be used in dire emergencies or when no operating room is available

3. Anesthesia:

   None

4. Equipment:
   a. Sterile prep solution
   b. Sterile gloves and towels
   c. 16 gauge or 18 gauge spinal needles

5. Positioning:

   Supine

6. Technique—Adults:

   Takes advantage of thin orbital roof.
   a. Sterile prep right conjunctiva and surrounding skin.
   b. With one hand, elevate eyelid and depress globe.
   c. Firmly hold spinal needle in other hand and penetrate anterior third of orbital roof 1–2 cm behind the orbital rim.
   d. Advance the needle toward an imaginary point intersecting coronal suture and midline. The frontal horn of ipsilateral ventricle lies at depth of 3–5 cm.
   e. Pull out stylet and observe for CSF. *If no CSF*, replace stylet and advance needle further 1–2 cm.
   f. *If still no CSF*, pull out the needle and re-aim trajectory slightly towards the midline.

7. Technique—Infants:

   Takes advantage of open fontanelle.
   a. Shave hair and sterile prep over fontanelle.

b. With the spinal needle, pierce the scalp and dura as far lateral as possible to prevent injury to superior sagittal sinus.

c. Advance needle 3–4 cm into ventricle.

d. Pull out stylet and observe for CSF. *If no CSF,* replace stylet and advance needle further 1 cm.

e. *If still no CSF,* pull out the needle and re-aim trajectory slightly towards the midline taking care not to pierce the superior sagittal sinus.

8. Complications and Management:
   a. Bleeding
      - If there is any change in neurologic exam, seizure, or unexpected blood seen after placement of the spinal needle, an immediate head CT should be obtained.
      - Most hemorrhages resolve spontaneously and require supportive care only.
      - In very rare circumstances operative evacuation of hematoma is indicated.
   b. Infection
      - The spinal needle should be removed as soon as possible and replaced by an IVC or other shunt if still needed.
   c. Tonsillar herniation
      - Can manifest as dilating unilateral pupil, change in mental status, Cushing's triad (hypertension, bradycardia, decreased respiratory rate).
      - Immediately remove the spinal needle.
      - Intubate and hyperventilation.
      - Mannitol (0.5–1 g/kg) and other diuretics
      - Emergent neurosurgery consult

E. SHUNT TAP

Ventriculo-peritoneal (V-P), ventriculo-atrial (V-A) and ventriculo-pleural shunts are commonly encountered neurosurgical devices used for chronic CSF diversion. A shunt tap is often required to evaluate for shunt problems.

1. Indications:
   a. Obtain CSF for analysis.
   b. Evaluate shunt function.
   c. Measure intraventricular pressure.
   d. Temporizing measure to remove CSF in a distally occluded shunt

    e. Injection of antibiotic or chemotherapeutic agents

    f. Injection of contrast agents

2. Contraindications:

    a. Scalp infection around shunt site

    b. Severe coagulopathy or platelets <25K

    c. Collapsed or slit ventricles

3. Anesthesia:

None usually needed

4. Equipment:

    a. Sterile prep solution

    b. Sterile gloves and towels

    c. 25 gauge or 23 gauge butterfly needles

    d. 10 mL syringe

    e. Manometer with stopcock

5. Positioning:

Supine

6. Technique:

    a. Palpate scalp for shunt bulb, which is usually in the right frontal or right occipital regions within 2 cm of the scalp incision used to insert the shunt. *Do not tamper* with other shunt components because it may affect shunt function (Fig. 5.17).

    b. Shave and prep the area for 5 minutes.

    c. Introduce the butterfly needle into bulb at a slight oblique angle and observe for spontaneous flow of CSF into tubing (Fig. 5.18).

    d. Attach stopcock with manometer to end of tubing, ensuring that the zero level on the manometer is level with the bulb.

    e. Measure the pressure, which represents the ventricular systemic pressure.

    f. Depress the distal occluder (if present) and measure manometer pressure. A slight rise in pressure indicates intact function of distal valve and shunt.

    g. Alternatively, depress proximal or inlet occluder (if present) and observe for distal run-off of CSF to evaluate distal shunt function.

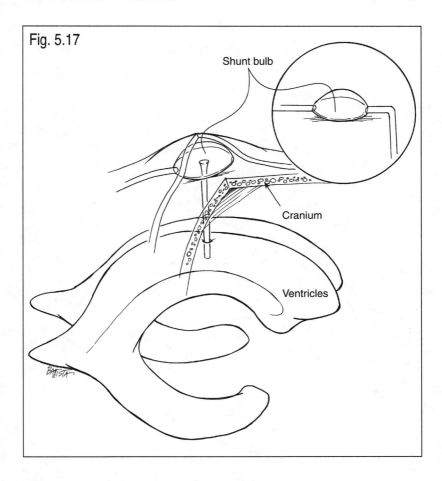

Fig. 5.17

Shunt bulb

Cranium

Ventricles

h. *If no spontaneous CSF flow* is observed, take 5 mL syringe and gently attempt to aspirate CSF. If CSF is aspirated easily, then the ventricular pressure is at or near zero. If CSF is difficult to aspirate or no CSF is obtained, then the proximal end of the shunt is occluded or the ventricles are collapsed, and aborting the procedure is necessary.

i. Send CSF for laboratory analysis.

j. Inject chemotherapeutic or antimicrobial agent if desired.

k. Withdraw needle and hold gentle pressure over bulb.

7. Complications and Management:

   a. Ventriculitis
      • Every time the shunt is manipulated, there is a chance of introducing infection into the system.

Fig. 5.18

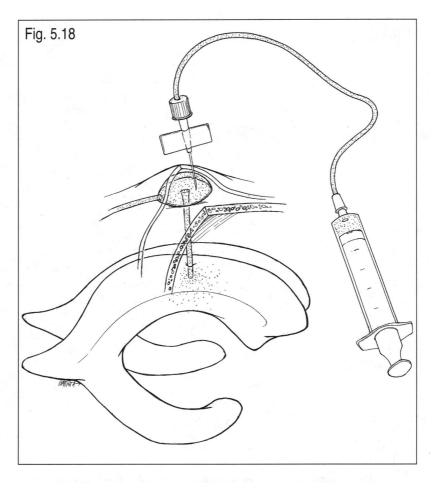

- In patients with systemic infection with no obvious CNS source, perform a lumbar puncture.
b. Occlusion
  - In patients with collapsed or slit-like ventricles, attempting to aspirate CSF can cause occlusion of the proximal shunt. A head CT prior to shunt tap can often avoid this complication.

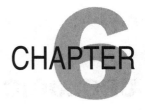

CHAPTER

UROLOGIC PROCEDURES

Author: Thomas J. Polascik, M.D.

UROLOGIC PROCEDURES

I. UROLOGY

The specialty of urology is concerned with the evaluation and treatment of various disorders and diseases of the male genitourinary tract and the female urinary tract. Although a broad spectrum of urologic disease is encountered daily in clinical practice, considerable effort is directed toward the medical and surgical treatment of voiding disorders. Quite often, the urologist encounters patients in acute urinary retention who are in need of timely intervention to relieve the obstruction.

A. URETHRAL CATHETERIZATION

1. Indications:
   a. Therapeutic:
      - Urinary retention
      - Urinary output monitoring
      - Irrigation of blood clots
      - Intravesical chemotherapy
      - Postoperative urethral stenting
   b. Diagnostic:
      - Collection of urine for studies
      - Retrograde instillation of contrast agents (cystourethrography)
      - Urodynamic studies

2. Contraindications:
   a. Acute prostatitis
   b. Suspected urethral disruption associated with blunt or pene-
      trating trauma
      • Blood at urethral meatus
      • Hemoscrotum (blood-filled scrotum)
      • Perineal ecchymoses
      • Nonpalpable prostate
      • Inability to void
   c. Severe urethral stricture

3. Anesthesia:
   None

4. Equipment:
   a. Urethral catheterization kit (includes Foley, povidone-iodine
      solution, lubricating jelly, 10 mL syringe, gloves, sterile tow-
      els, and urinary drainage bag)
   b. Recommend 18 fr Foley for males and 16 fr for females.

5. Positioning:
   Supine (men), frog-leg (women).

6. Technique—Catheterization of Men:
   a. Place sterile towels around the penis (Fig. 6.1).
   b. Retract the foreskin (if present). Grasp the penis laterally
      with the nondominant hand and place it on maximum
      stretch *perpendicular* to the body to straighten the anterior
      urethra.
   c. Swab the glans with povidone-iodine with the dominant
      hand. Observe sterile technique at all times.
   d. Lubricate the catheter with lubricating jelly and grasp with
      the dominant hand. It is often helpful to inject 10 mL water
      soluble jelly (or 2% lidocaine jelly) into the urethra prior to
      passing the catheter (Fig. 6.2).
   e. Using steady, gentle pressure, advance the catheter into the
      urethra until both the hub of the catheter is reached and urine
      is returned. Inflate the balloon with 10 mL normal saline.
   f. If urine is not returned, irrigate the catheter to confirm cor-
      rect placement prior to inflating the balloon.

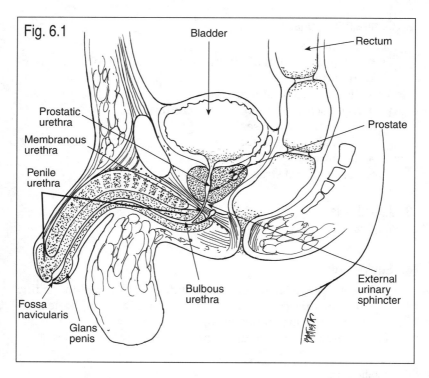

Fig. 6.1

g. *Replace the foreskin.* Connect the catheter to a urinary drainage bag.

h. If the catheter cannot be easily passed, a strategy for successful catheterization must be planned.

7. Strategies for Difficult Catheterization of Men:

If resistance is met during catheter advancement, manually palpate the catheter tip to define the point of obstruction along the urethra (Fig. 6.3). Once the location and nature of the lesion is defined, the next step is to develop a strategy for bypassing the obstruction.

a. Anterior urethral obstruction—urethral stricture, a concentric narrowing of the lumen by scar tissue. Can occur at the fossa navicularis, bulbous urethra, or along the penile urethra.

   • Etiology: sexually transmitted disease, prior urethral instrumentation including transurethral prostatic resection (TURP), trauma.

   • Signs/symptoms: splayed and/or slow stream, straining.

   • Strategy—penile urethral stricture: (1) Use 16 fr or smaller

Fig. 6.2

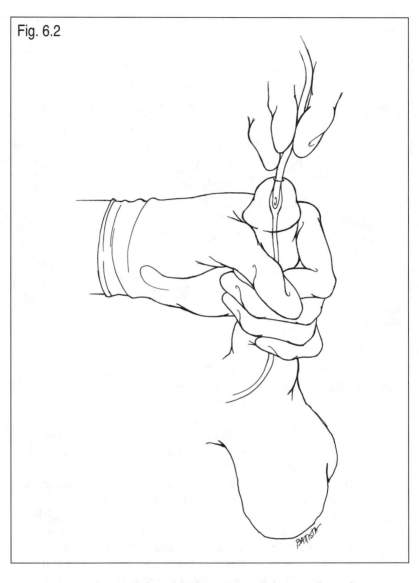

straight-tip Foley. (2) If unsuccessful, consult urology to attempt catheter placement.
- Strategy—bulbar urethral stricture: (1) Same as above. (2) If unsuccessful, 16 fr *Coude-tip* will better negotiate the natural angle of the bulbomembranous junction. A *Coude catheter* has a curved-tip that enables one to better engage the normal S-shaped curve of the bulbomembranous junction or to bypass an enlarged, obstructing prostate in the

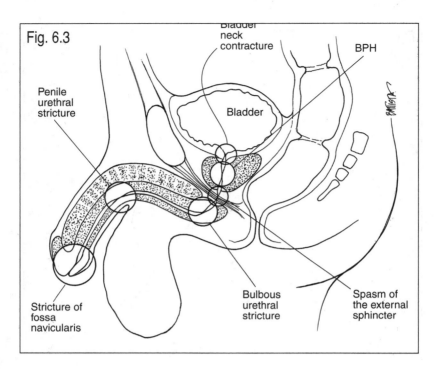

Fig. 6.3

Bladder neck contracture

BPH

Penile urethral stricture

Bladder

Stricture of fossa navicularis

Bulbous urethral stricture

Spasm of the external sphincter

male urethra. To insert a Coude catheter, always keep the angled tip pointing *superiorly* and follow steps *6a–h*.

b. Posterior urethral obstructions
   • Spasm of the external urinary sphincter
      (1) Etiology: contraction of the voluntary sphincter secondary to anxiety or pain. *Often the cause of unsuccessful catheterization of men <50 years old.*
      (2) Signs: as the catheter tip approaches the sphincter, the patient becomes tense and complains of pain.
      (3) Strategy: (a) Inject 10 mL of lubricant (water soluble jelly works as well as 2% lidocaine jelly). (b) After reaching the sphincter, pull the catheter back a few centimeters. (c) Distract the patient with conversation and by having him breathe deeply. (d) Advance the Foley steadily when the patient is relaxed.
   • Benign prostatic hypertrophy (BPH)
      (1) Suspect with age >60, prior TURP, treatment with finasteride (Proscar) or terazosin (Hytrin).
      (2) Symptoms: hesitancy, intermittent and/or slow stream, straining, sensation of incomplete emptying.
      (3) Strategy: (a) A large catheter (18 fr or 20 fr) provides

the additional stiffness needed to overcome the obstruction. A Coude-tip is often helpful to negotiate the
angle between the bulbous and membranous urethra.
(b) Use the *two-person technique:* while catheter placement is attempted in the usual fashion, the assistant
places a lubricated index finger in the rectum and pal-
pates the apex of the prostate. The tip of the catheter
can usually be felt just distal to the apex (Fig. 6.4).

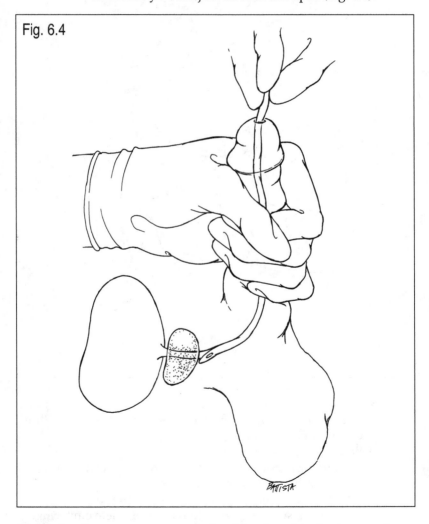

Fig. 6.4

The index finger presses anteriorly, thus elevating the apex and
straightening out the area of obstruction (Fig. 6.5).

Fig. 6.5

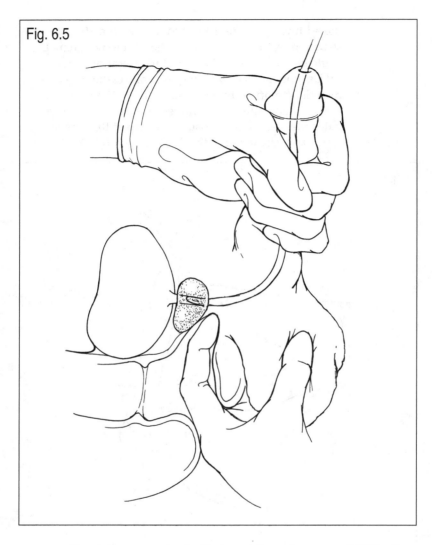

- Prostate cancer: typically is not the sole cause of difficult catheterization unless the cancer is locally advanced. Strategy is similar to BPH.
- Bladder neck contracture
  (1) Etiology: prior open or radical retropubic prostatectomy, bladder neck incision or TURP.
  (2) Symptoms: hesitancy, intermittent and/or slow stream, straining, sensation of incomplete emptying.
  (3) Strategy: (a) Attempt a 16 fr Coude following steps 6a–h. (b) Consult urology.

8. Technique—Catheterization of Women:

a. Place patient in a frog-leg position (Fig. 6.6).

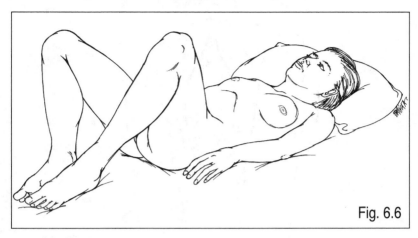

Fig. 6.6

Alternatively, for women who are unable to abduct the thighs, flexion at the hips provides easy access to the urethra.

b. Place sterile towels around the introitus.

c. Use the nondominant hand to spread apart labia minora (Fig. 6.7).

d. Use the dominant hand to swab the urethral meatus with sterile prep solution.

e. Using sterile technique, grasp a lubricated 16 fr catheter with the dominant hand and advance it approximately 10 cm through the urethral meatus or until urine is returned.

f. Inflate the balloon with 10 mL normal saline.

g. Attach the catheter to the urinary drainage bag.

h. If the urethral meatus cannot be easily located, place the patient in the dorsal lithotomy position and have a bright examination light available.

i. *The urethral meatus may still be difficult to visualize* due to vaginal atrophy, congenital female hypospadias, or a prior surgical procedure that has altered the location of the meatus. In these instances, the meatus is typically located deeper within the vaginal vault and anteriorly in the urethrovaginal septum.

j. A vaginal speculum may be helpful to locate the meatus.

k. Confirmation of correct catheter position can be accomplished by placing a lubricated index finger in the vagina and palpating the catheter anteriorly through the urethrovaginal septum.

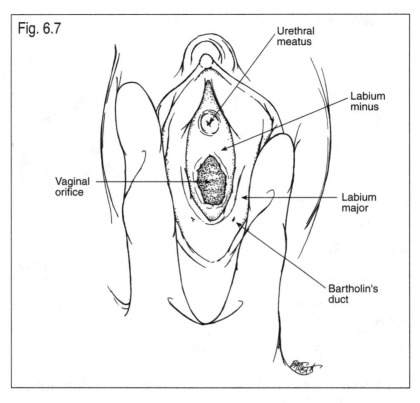

Fig. 6.7

Urethral meatus

Labium minus

Vaginal orifice

Labium major

Bartholin's duct

9. Complications and Management:
   a. Suspicion of false passage
      • Best evaluated by cystoscopy.
      • Abort further attempts and consult urology.
   b. Relief of acute retention: It is usually safe to drain the entire bladder contents rapidly. Observe the patient for post-obstructive diuresis. If the urine output is >200 mL/hr over the next several hours or if patient has other comorbid diseases (i.e., congestive heart failure, azotemia, sepsis), consider admitting.
   c. Hypotension
      • Early hypotension is typically a vasovagal response to the acute relief of a distended bladder.
      • Late hypotension can occur from excessive post-obstructive diuresis.
   d. Hematuria
      • Caused by traumatic catheter placement or by small mucosal disruptions following the acute relief of a distended bladder.

- Treat with fluids, catheter irrigation, and monitoring.
  e. Paraphimosis
  - See Section D in this chapter for treatment.

B. PERCUTANEOUS SUPRAPUBIC CYSTOSTOMY

There are two main types of percutaneous suprapubic catheters used: Bonanno percutaneous suprapubic catheter set (Becton-Dickinson and Co., Rutherford, NJ) or Stamey percutaneous suprapubic catheter set in 10, 12, or 14 fr (Cook Urological, Spencer, IA). The technique of insertion differs depending on which type is used.

1. Indications:
   a. Urethral stricture
   b. False passage
   c. Inability to catheterize
   d. Acute prostatitis
   e. Traumatic urethral disruption
   f. Periurethral abscess

2. Contraindications:
   a. Prior midline infraumbilical incision
   b. *Nondistended bladder*
   c. Coagulopathy
   d. Pregnancy
   e. Carcinoma of the bladder
   f. Pelvic irradiation

3. Anesthesia:
   1% lidocaine

4. Equipment:
   a. Bonanno percutaneous suprapubic catheter set or Stamey percutaneous suprapubic catheter set in 10, 12, or 14 fr
   b. Urinary drainage bag
   c. Sterile prep solution
   d. Sterile gloves and towels
   e. 20 gauge spinal needle
   f. 10 mL syringes (2)
   g. 22–25 gauge needles
   h. 3–0 nylon suture

    i. Needle driver
    j. Suture scissors
    k. Safety razor

5. Positioning:

Supine

6. Technique—Bonanno Catheter:

    a. *Administer appropriate antibiotics*, especially if urinary tract infection is suspected.
    b. Percuss the suprapubic area to confirm an adequately distended bladder.
    c. Shave, prep, and drape the suprapubic area.
    d. Place the disposable catheter sleeve adjacent to the suture disc (Fig. 6.8).

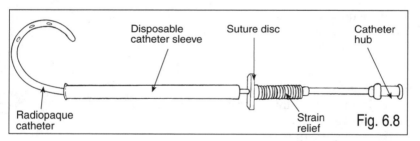

Fig. 6.8

Insert the 18 gauge puncture needle into the catheter so that the needle tip is always directed along the inside of the curve. To prevent the needle tip from damaging the inside of the catheter during assembly, advance the needle and the catheter sleeve simultaneously (the catheter sleeve straightens the "J" of the distal catheter), always maintaining the needle tip within the center of the catheter sleeve (Fig. 6.9).

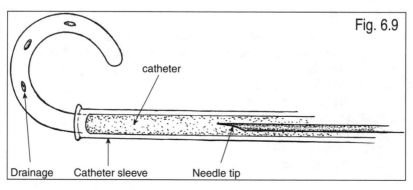

Fig. 6.9

e. Once the bevel of the needle extends beyond the end of the catheter, remove the disposable catheter sleeve and rotate the pink needle hub clockwise to lock the needle to the catheter hub.

f. If catheter damage occurs during assembly, *discard the catheter*.

g. Anesthetize the skin with 1% lidocaine at a point 2 finger-breadths above the symphysis pubis in the midline (Fig. 6.10).

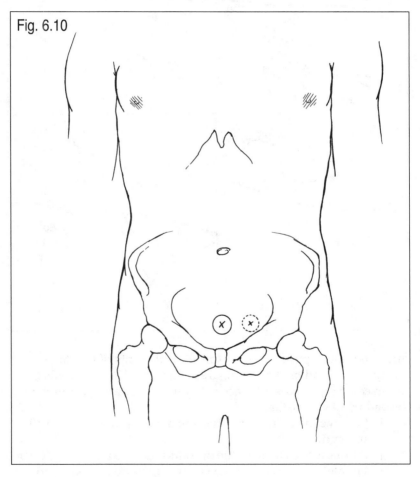

Fig. 6.10

If the patient has a previous midline incision scar, anesthetize 2 finger-breadths above the pubic symphysis and 2 cm lateral to the incision. Direct the angle of the needle 60° to the skin and aim inferomedially toward the symphysis. Real-time ultrasonography can be helpful.

h. Insert the spinal needle into the anesthetized skin 2 finger-breadths above the pubic symphysis in the midline (also 2 cm lateral to the midline if an old midline incision scar is present). Direct the needle toward the symphysis, using a *60° angle to the skin* (Fig. 6.11).

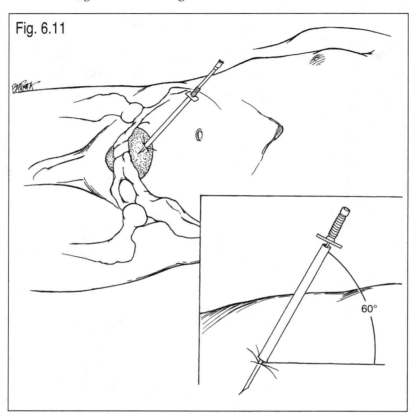

Fig. 6.11

After the skin is punctured, two additional points of resistance (rectus fascia and bladder wall) are encountered as the needle is advanced. Stop needle advancement after penetrating through the second point of resistance.

    i. Remove the obturator of the spinal needle and attach a 10 mL syringe.

    j. If *urine is not aspirated,* the obturator of the spinal needle can be safely replaced and the needle can be advanced up to one centimeter at a time until urine is aspirated.

    k. If *urine is aspirated,* leave the needle in place as a guide.

    l. Next, take the previously assembled suprapubic catheter and puncture the skin adjacent to the spinal needle. Advance the suprapubic catheter in a similar manner as described above (step h), following the tract of the spinal needle. The catheter has a reference mark on the needle obturator indicating the distance at which the catheter should have penetrated the bladder in most patients.

m. Remove the black vent plug, attach a 10 mL syringe to the catheter hub, and aspirate.

n. *Caution:* Be certain to remove the black vent plug when checking position and not the needle (pink hub). *Once the needle has been withdrawn from a suprapubic catheter, do not reinsert it!* Remove the entire device from the patient and reassemble as in step d.

o. Once urine is obtained, advance the catheter an additional 1–2 cm.

p. To disengage the suprapubic catheter and the needle obturator, stabilize the catheter and rotate the pink hub of the needle obturator *counterclockwise.*

q. *Stabilize the needle while advancing the catheter* over it until the suture disc lies flush with the skin.

r. Aspirate again to confirm proper catheter placement. Insert the connecting tube between the catheter and the urinary drainage bag.

s. Secure the catheter to the skin with 3–0 nylon suture. Tape the catheter to the abdominal wall to avoid kinking the tubing.

7. Technique—Stamey Catheter:

a. *Administer appropriate antibiotics,* especially if urinary tract infection is suspected.

b. Percuss the suprapubic area to confirm an adequately distended bladder.

c. Shave, prep, and drape the suprapubic area.

d. Guide the needle obturator into the catheter tip to stretch and straighten the self-retaining mechanism of the Malecot catheter. Secure its position with the Luer lock to close the Malecot wings (Fig. 6.12).

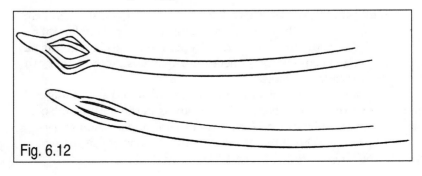

Fig. 6.12

  e. If catheter damage occurs during assembly, *discard the catheter*.

  f. Anesthetize the skin with 1% lidocaine 2 fingerbreadths above the symphysis pubis in the midline (Fig. 6.13).

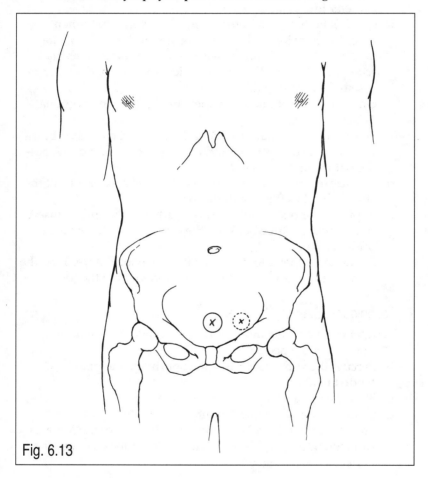

Fig. 6.13

If the patient has a previous midline incision scar, anesthetize 2 fingerbreadths above the pubic symphysis and 2 cm lateral to the incision. Infiltrating the deeper rectus fascia with the 22 gauge needle becomes necessary when using the larger calibre Stamey catheter.

  g. Insert the spinal needle into the anesthetized skin 2 fingerbreadths above the pubic symphysis in the midline (also 2 cm lateral to the midline if an old midline incision scar is present). Direct the needle toward the symphysis, using a *60° angle to the skin* (Fig. 6.14).

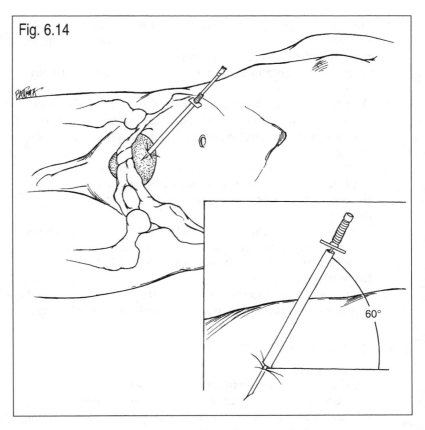

Fig. 6.14

60°

After the skin is punctured, two additional points of resistance (rectus fascia and bladder wall) are encountered as the needle is advanced. Stop needle advancement after penetrating through the second point of resistance.

    h. Remove the obturator of the spinal needle and attach a 10 mL syringe.

    i. If *urine is not aspirated,* the obturator of the spinal needle can be safely replaced and the needle can be advanced up to one centimeter at a time until urine is aspirated.

    j. If *urine is aspirated,* leave the needle in place as a guide.

    k. Next, take the previously assembled suprapubic catheter and puncture the skin adjacent to the spinal needle. Advance the suprapubic catheter in a similar manner as described above (step g), following the tract of the spinal needle. The catheter has a reference mark on the needle obturator indicating the distance at which the catheter should have penetrated the bladder in most patients.

    l. Attach a 10 mL syringe to the catheter hub and aspirate.

m. *Caution: If the needle is mistakenly withdrawn from a suprapubic catheter, do not reinsert it!* Remove the entire device from the patient and reassemble as in step d.
n. Once urine is obtained, advance the catheter an additional 1–2 cm.
o. To disengage the suprapubic catheter and the needle obturator, stabilize the catheter and rotate the white hub of the needle obturator *counterclockwise.* This maneuver opens the Malecot wings.
p. *Withdraw the needle obturator while stabilizing the catheter.*
q. Aspirate again to confirm proper catheter placement. Insert the connecting tube between the catheter and the urinary drainage bag.
r. Slowly withdraw the catheter until the Malecot wings meet the resistance of the bladder wall. Then, advance the catheter approximately 2 cm back into the bladder to allow for movement.
s. Secure the catheter to the skin with 3–0 nylon suture. Tape the catheter to the abdominal wall to avoid kinking the tubing.

8. Complications and Management:

a. Bowel injury
  • If the bladder is not sufficiently distended, there is increased risk of entering the peritoneum or the rectum.
  • If bowel is entered, one may exchange the needle and continue with the procedure. Peritonitis is rare.
b. Hematuria/clots
  • If obstruction of the catheter from clots is suspected, gently irrigate the suprapubic catheter with normal saline. These percutaneous cystostomy catheters are of small calibre (14 gauge lumen Bonanno; 10–14 fr Stamey) and are often insufficient for treating gross hematuria with clot obstruction.
  • Leakage around the insertion site may indicate catheter damage or obstruction.
  • Urology consult

C. PENILE NERVE BLOCK

1. Indications:

To anesthetize the penis for:
a. Reduction of paraphimosis

b. Circumcision
c. Dorsal slit

2. Contraindications:

Uncorrectable coagulopathy

3. Anesthesia:

1% lidocaine. *Avoid epinephrine.*

4. Equipment:

a. Sterile prep solution
b. Sterile gloves and towels
c. 10 mL syringe
d. 22 gauge needle

5. Positioning:

Supine

6. Technique:

a. Prep and drape the suprapubic skin, penis, and anterolateral scrotum.
b. Identify the penopubic junction.
c. Using a 22 gauge needle on a syringe filled with 1% plain lidocaine, puncture the skin 1 cm cranial to the penopubic junction near the lateral border of the penis on the patient's right side (Fig. 6.15).

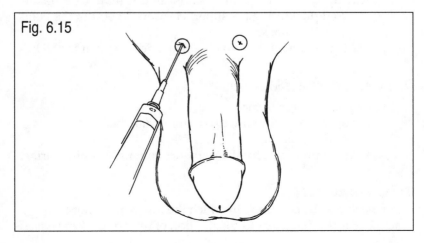

Fig. 6.15

d. Advance the needle until the needle tip penetrates through the subtle resistance of Buck's fascia (Fig. 6.16).

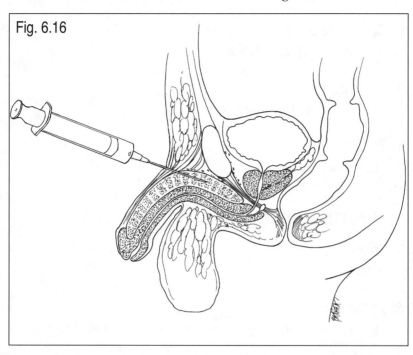

Fig. 6.16

e. Gently aspirate to prevent intravascular injection prior to injecting 5 mL 1% plain lidocaine just beneath Buck's fascia.
f. Repeat the same sequence on the patient's left side.
g. At the base of the penis, circumferentially infiltrate the skin with approximately 5 mL 1% lidocaine. Care must be taken to avoid puncturing the superficial dorsal veins of the penis and their tributaries.
h. Wait at least 5 minutes to obtain an adequate penile block.

7. Complications and Management:
   a. Expanding hematoma
      • Apply direct pressure to control hemorrhage.
   b. Penile ischemia
      • Avoid premixed local anesthetics containing epinephrine.

D. DORSAL SLIT

Phimosis is the condition in which the foreskin cannot be retracted over the glans due to constriction of the orifice. *Paraphimosis* is the condition in which the foreskin, once retracted proximal to the glans, cannot be replaced to its normal position. The foreskin is edematous and tender when paraphimosis exists. With an adequate penile block, paraphimosis can be manually reduced in most circumstances by compressing the glans for 5–10 minutes to reduce the edema, followed by pulling the foreskin over the glans with the two-handed technique. Additionally, a dorsal slit can be difficult to properly perform with paraphimosis (Fig. 6.17).

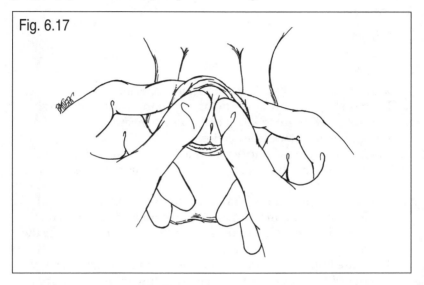

Fig. 6.17

1. Indications:
   a. Unreducible paraphimosis
   b. Severe phimosis associated with acute or recurrent infections (balanitis, urethritis)
   c. Voiding difficulty or inability to catheterize

2. Contraindications:

   No absolute contraindications

3. Anesthesia:

   Penile block

4. Equipment:
   a. Sterile prep solution
   b. Sterile gloves and towels

    c. Straight clamps (2)
    d. Scissors
    e. Needle driver
    f. 4–0 chromic sutures
    g. 10 mL syringe
    h. 22 gauge needle
    i. 1% lidocaine

5. Positioning:

Supine

6. Technique:

a. Administer antibiotics if infection is present.
b. Sterilely prep and drape penis, pre-symphysis, and anterior scrotum. Be sure to adequately prep beneath foreskin.
c. Place penile block (see Section C).
d. Place a straight clamp across the dorsal surface of the foreskin in the midline, carefully avoiding injury to the glans (Fig. 6.18).
e. After clamping for one minute, remove the clamp and cut along the crimp mark. Adequate length of incision is confirmed by the ability of the foreskin to easily retract over the glans.
f. Suture both sides with running 4–0 chromic beginning at the apex of the incision and progressing toward the distal foreskin. Both the mucosal and serosal skin edges must always be visualized and incorporated into the closure when suturing the wound (Fig. 6.19).
g. Dress with sterile gauze.

7. Complications and Management:

a. Bleeding
    • The crushing straight clamp should minimize bleeding during the procedure.
    • Apply direct pressure on any bleeding point and oversew if necessary.
    • If bleeding persists, an Elastoplast dressing should tamponade it. Do not apply the dressing too tightly in order to minimize distal glanular ischemia.
b. Infection
    • Local wound care
    • Antibiotics.

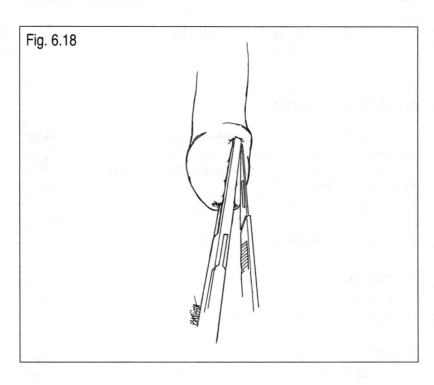

Fig. 6.18

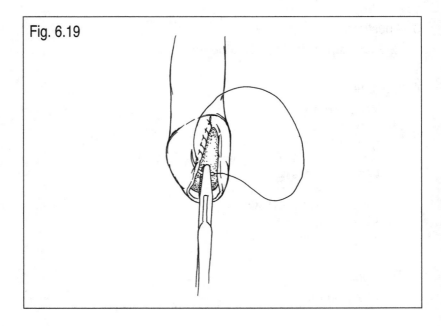

Fig. 6.19

　　c. Urethral injury or injury to the glans
　　　• Urology consult

II. GYNECOLOGY

　　Gynecology is concerned with the evaluation and treatment of various disorders and diseases of the female reproductive tract, as well as its normal physiologic function. Culdocentesis and surgical drainage of a Bartholin's abscess are two common bedside procedures performed in clinical practice.

A. CULDOCENTESIS

1. Indications:
　　a. Suspected pelvic abscess
　　b. Possible ectopic pregnancy

2. Contraindications:
　　a. Obliterated cul-de-sac
　　b. Severely retroverted uterus

3. Anesthesia:
　　2% lidocaine jelly, 1% lidocaine solution

4. Equipment:
　　a. Sterile prep solution
　　b. Gloves
　　c. Speculum
　　d. Single-tooth tenaculum or sponge forceps
　　e. 10 mL syringes (2)
　　f. 20 or 22 gauge spinal needle
　　g. Long cotton-tipped swabs
　　h. Kelly clamp
　　i. Scalpel on long handle

5. Positioning:
　　Dorsal lithotomy

6. Technique:

a. Swab the introitus with sterile prep solution.

b. Insert the speculum. If the posterior cul-de-sac is not fully prepared, use the long cotton-tipped swabs to complete the prep. The posterior cul-de-sac will be bulging or tender if an abscess is present (Fig. 6.20).

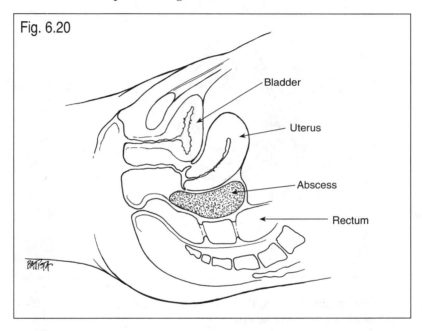

Fig. 6.20

- Bladder
- Uterus
- Abscess
- Rectum

c. Place a long cotton-tipped swab generously lubricated with 2% lidocaine jelly on the midline posterior vaginal wall 2 cm below the cervix. Wait a few minutes for adequate anesthesia.

d. The posterior lip of the cervix can be gently grasped with a sponge forceps and elevated. Alternatively, infiltrate the posterior cervical lip with 2–3 mL of 1% lidocaine and, once anesthetized, cautiously apply a single-tooth tenaculum. Elevate the cervix (Fig. 6.21).

e. With the spinal needle mounted on the 10 mL syringe, insert the needle tip through the anesthetized midline posterior vaginal wall into the cul-de-sac and aspirate (Fig. 6.22).

f. The presence of blood or pus confirms the diagnosis. If fluid cannot be withdrawn, reposition the needle. Send fluid for culture and/or analysis as indicated.

g. If an abscess (pus) is encountered, it must be fully incised

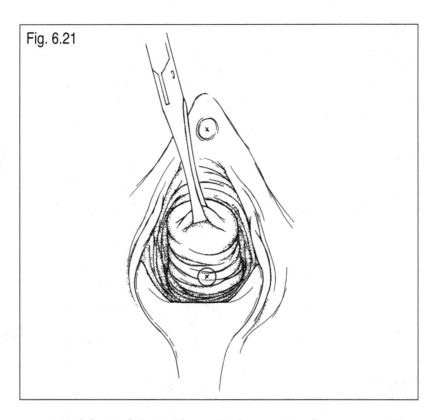

Fig. 6.21

and drained. Incise the vaginal mucosa at the puncture site with a #15 or #11 scalpel.

h. Bluntly spread with a Kelly clamp and express the pus (Fig. 6.23).

i. Irrigate until the abscess cavity is clear.

j. If no fluid is aspirated, it is difficult to unequivocally rule-out an abscess or fluid collection in the cul-de-sac. Sonography can be helpful in select cases.

7. Complications and Management:

a. Bleeding
   • Apply direct pressure on the bleeding site with the long cotton-tipped swab.

B. INCISION AND DRAINAGE OF BARTHOLIN'S ABSCESS

A Bartholin's cyst results from inspissation of the drainage duct and presents as a unilateral swelling lateral to the posterior

Fig. 6.22

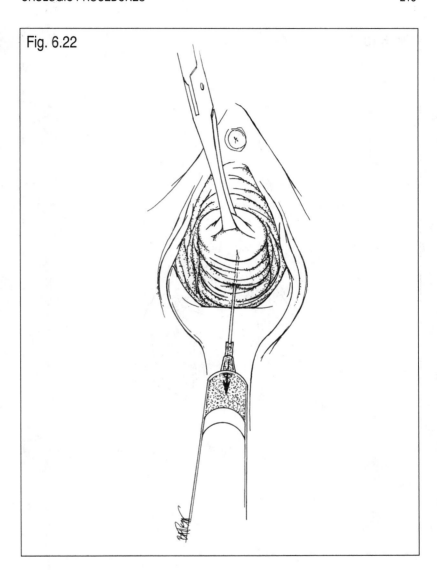

fourchette. Bartholin's cysts are usually 2 cm in diameter and are asymptomatic. However, these cysts can become quite painful if secondarily infected.

1. Indications:
   a. Relief of symptoms
   b. Failure to respond to conservative medical management

Fig. 6.23

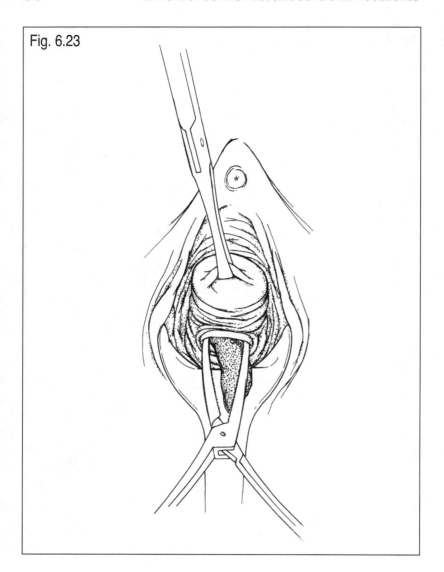

2. Contraindications:

Non-fluctuant cyst/abscess

3. Anesthesia:

Fluro Ethyl (Gebauer Pharmaceutical, Cleveland, OH) topical anesthetic spray

4. Equipment:

a. Sterile prep solution
b. Sterile towels and gloves
c. #15 scalpel
d. Kelly clamp
e. 10 mL syringe
f. Word Bartholin Gland Catheter (TFX Medical, Duluth, GA)
g. Saline irrigation
h. NuGauze packing

5. Positioning:

Dorsal lithotomy

6. Technique:

a. Administer antibiotics if indicated.
b. Examination should reveal a fluctuant, ripened abscess. Prep and drape.
c. *If cyst is not yet fluctuant,* management consists of Sitz baths, antibiotics, and analgesics. Drainage is indicated when fluctuant.
d. The abscess is approached medially through the mucosa of the vagina. Carefully spray Fluro Ethyl topical anesthetic over the puncture site only.
e. A 1–2 cm incision through the vaginal mucosa into the abscess cavity is sufficient for drainage (Fig. 6.24). Manually (or with a Kelly clamp) express all of the pus and copiously irrigate the abscess cavity with normal saline. The cavity is then packed with NuGauze dressing.
f. Alternatively, a Word Bartholin Gland Catheter can be used. This is a 5 cm, 10 fr catheter that is inserted through a 1–2 mm stab incision into the abscess cavity after it has been irrigated. Inflate the 5 mL balloon with normal saline. The catheter does not need to be further secured to the introitus.
g. Send fluid for culture.

7. Complications and Management:

a. Bleeding
  • Apply direct pressure.
  • If not successful, packing the cavity with NuGauze should stop the bleeding.

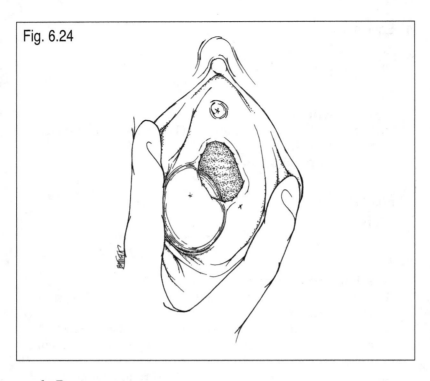

Fig. 6.24

b. Recurrence
   - Should be avoidable by initially providing complete drainage of the abscess followed by daily packing changes.
   - Elective operative marsupialization should prevent recurrence.

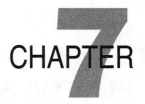

CHAPTER 7

PLASTIC SURGERY AND HAND PROCEDURES

Author: Bernadette H. Wang, M.D.

I. Regional Anesthesia
- A. Local/Field Block
- B. Digital Block
- C. Wrist Block

II. Tourniquets
- A. Finger Tourniquet
- B. Arm Tourniquet

III. Hand Procedures
- A. Removal of a Nail
- B. Repair of Nailbed Laceration
- C. Drainage of Subungal Hematoma
- D. Treatment of Paronychia
- E. Incision and Drainage of Upper Extremity Abscess

IV. Complex Lacerations
- A. Lip
- B. Ear

PLASTIC SURGERY AND HAND PROCEDURES

Plastic surgery is a specialty devoted to managing difficult wounds, with the goal of restoring function and creating the best aesthetic outcome. Plastic surgical procedures involve the appropriate use of regional anesthesia and tourniquets when managing wounds in areas of important form and function, such as the face and the hand.

I. REGIONAL ANESTHESIA

Local anesthetics work by producing nerve conduction blockade at the level of nerve membrane receptors. The most commonly used agent is lidocaine. Addition of epinephrine (epi) reduces bleeding and systemic absorption by local vasoconstriction. The toxic limit of lidocaine is 5 mg/kg without epinephrine and 7 mg/kg with epinephrine. (Note that 1% lidocaine contains 10 mg/ml.) Other local anesthetics are shown below:

Local Anesthetic	Onset	Maximum dose (mg/kg)		Duration of action (hrs)	
		plain	with epi	plain	with epi
Bupivacaine (Marcaine)	slow	2.5	3.5	2.0–4.0	4.0–8.0
Lidocaine (Xylocaine)	rapid	5.0	7.0	0.5–2.0	1.0–4.0
Procaine (Novocaine)	slow	6.0	9.0	0.25–0.5	0.5–1.0
Tetracaine (Pontocaine)	slow	1.5	2.5	2.0–3.0	2.0–4.0

A. LOCAL/FIELD BLOCK

1. Indications:

   Anesthesia for:
   a. Surgical procedures
   b. Wounds that require irrigation, débridement, and/or repair

2. Contraindications:

   a. None when using local anesthetics without epinephrine.
   b. Epinephrine should not be used at anatomic sites supplied
      by end-arteries (fingers, toes, nose, ears, penis) or in infec-
      tion-prone wounds (animal or human bites, contaminated
      wounds).

3. Anesthesia:

   Choose from the chart above.

4. Equipment:

   a. Sterile prep solution
   b. Sterile gloves and towels
   c. 25 gauge needle
   d. 10 mL syringe

5. Positioning:

   Varies with location of wound.

6. Technique:

   a. Sterile prep and drape area of interest.
   b. Stretch skin taut to facilitate penetration and directly infil-
      trate local anesthetic through wound edges and inside
      wound with a 25 gauge needle (Fig. 7.1).
   c. Inject the anesthetic slowly or add $NaHCO_3$ (1 ml 10%
      $NaHCO_3$ to 9 ml 1% lidocaine) to reduce pain on infiltration.
      If more $NaHCO_3$ is added, it will precipitate in the lido-
      caine. If this occurs, *do not use the solution.*

7. Complications and Management:

   a. Intravascular injection or overdose
      • Initial signs of toxicity include dizziness, restlessness,

Fig. 7.1

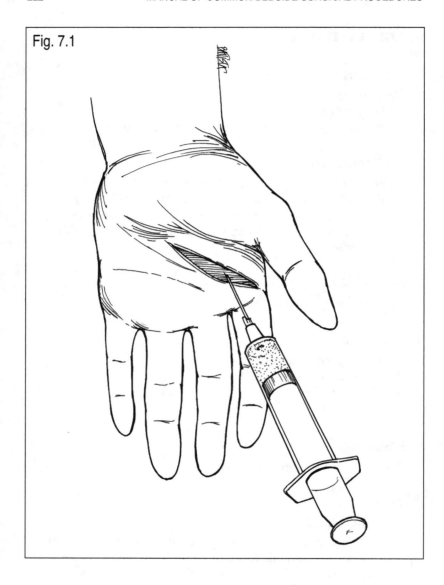

paresthesias, twitching, and may lead to generalized
seizures and cardiovascular collapse.
- Stop the local anesthetic and hyperventilate with 100%
  O_2.
- Use IV diazepam (0.1–0.3 mg/kg) for seizures.
- Initiate ACLS protocols if necessary. Prolonged CPR is indicated because the effects of the anesthetic will subside as
  the drug redistributes.

B. DIGITAL BLOCK

1. Indications:

   Wounds involving the fingers or thumb

2. Contraindications:

   Injury to the digital neurovascular bundle

3. Anesthesia:

   Agents that lack epinephrine. (See chart in Section I.)

4. Equipment:

   a. Sterile prep solution
   b. Sterile gloves and towels
   c. 3/4 inch 25 gauge needle
   d. 10 mL syringe

5. Positioning:

   Supine with arm extended on an arm board

6. Technique:

   a. Sterile prep and drape fingers and web spaces.
   b. Using a 3/4 inch 25 gauge needle, puncture the skin in the two
      surrounding interdigital web spaces and advance the needle
      parallel to the horizontal plane of the hand and fingers (Fig. 7.2).
   c. With the full length of the needle in the web space, aspirate
      to make sure needle is *not intravascular* and then inject *each of
      the two surrounding interdigital web spaces* with 3 mL 1% lido-
      caine as shown in the diagram (Fig. 7.3).
   d. If blocking *the thumb,* the digital nerves are located more
      volarly so the needle must be aimed more volarly as well.
   e. Infiltrate another 3 mL 1% lidocaine at the dorsum of the
      metacarpophalangeal joint (knuckle) to block the dorsal
      branches of the radial digital nerve. Avoid circumferential
      block at base.
   f. Allow at least 5 minutes for the onset of anesthesia depend-
      ing on the agent. If a *total block is not achieved* in about 20–30
      minutes, then an additional 2 mL may be administered in
      each web space.

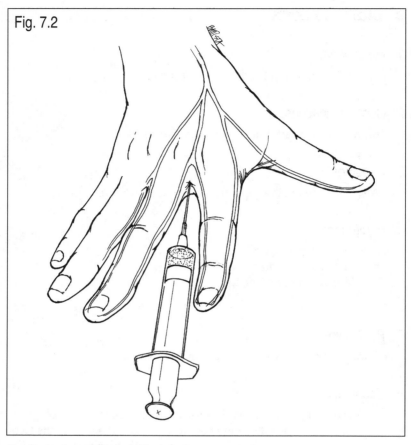

Fig. 7.2

7. Complications and Management:

a. Intravascular injection or overdose
   - Initial signs of toxicity include dizziness, restlessness, paresthesias, twitching, and may lead to generalized seizures and cardiovascular collapse.
   - Stop the local anesthetic and hyperventilate with 100% O_2.
   - Use IV diazepam (0.1–0.3 mg/kg) for seizures.
   - Initiate ACLS protocols if necessary. Prolonged CPR is indicated because the effects of the anesthetic will subside as the drug redistributes.

C. WRIST BLOCK

1. Indications:

Complex hand wounds

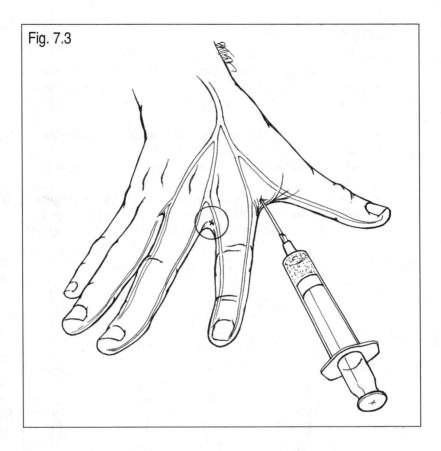

Fig. 7.3

2. Contraindications:

Injury to median/radial/ulnar nerves and vessels

3. Anesthesia:

See chart in Section I. Recommend 2% lidocaine.

4. Equipment:

a. Sterile prep solution
b. Sterile gloves and towels
c. 25 gauge needle
d. 10 mL syringe

5. Positioning:

Supine with arm extended on arm board

6. Technique:

a. Sterile prep and drape wrist and hand.

b. Using a 25 gauge needle, inject each of the following 4 sites with 5 mL 2% lidocaine. Be careful not to elicit paresthesias. *Always aspirate* before injection to avoid intravascular injection.

- Median nerve: (1) Locate palmaris longus by thumb-5th finger opposition and wrist flexion. (2) Inject anesthetic radial to palmaris longus at the level of the wrist flexion crease.
- Ulnar nerve: (1) Locate flexor carpi ulnaris by 5th finger abduction and wrist flexion. (2) Inject anesthetic radial to flexor carpi ulnaris at level of wrist flexion crease (Fig. 7.4).

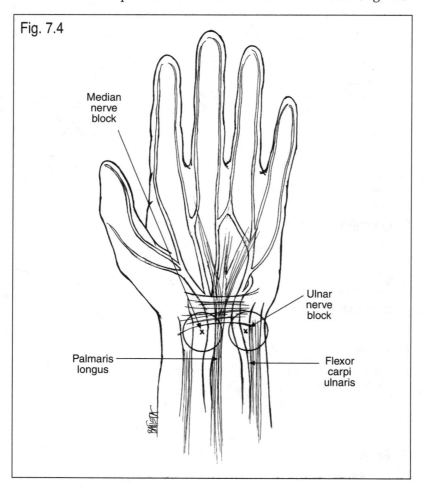

Fig. 7.4

- Radial nerve: (1) Accentuate the borders of the anatomic snuff box by thumb abduction. (2) Inject anesthetic over the radial styloid at the base of the snuff box.
- Dorsal cutaneous branch of the ulnar nerve: Inject anesthetic over the ulnar styloid prominence (Fig. 7.5).

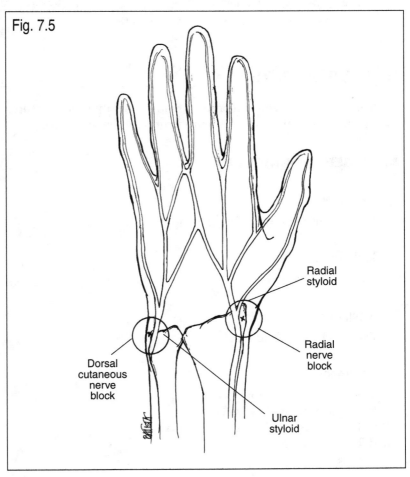

Fig. 7.5

Radial styloid

Radial nerve block

Dorsal cutaneous nerve block

Ulnar styloid

7. Complications and Management:

a. Intravascular injection or overdose
- Initial signs of toxicity include dizziness, restlessness, paresthesias, twitching, and may lead to generalized seizures and cardiovascular collapse.
- Stop the local anesthetic and hyperventilate with 100% O_2.
- Use IV diazepam (0.1–0.3 mg/kg) for seizures.

- Initiate ACLS protocols if necessary. Prolonged CPR is indicated because the effects of the anesthetic will subside as the drug redistributes.
  b. Paresthesias
    - Stop injection.
    - Advance or pull back needle to move a few millimeters away from nerve and reinject anesthetic.

II. TOURNIQUETS

Tourniquets provide a bloodless field so that injured structures can be identified safely and uninjured parts can be protected.

A. FINGER TOURNIQUET

1. Indications:

   Wounds involving the finger or thumb

2. Contraindications:

   None

3. Anesthesia:

   Digital block or field block

4. Equipment:

   a. Sterile prep solution
   b. Sterile gloves and towels
   c. 1/4 inch or 1/2 inch sterile Penrose drain
   d. Halsted clamp
   e. Scissors

5. Positioning:

   Supine with arm extended on arm board

6. Technique:

   a. Sterile prep and drape finger.
   b. Wrap finger tightly with a Penrose drain starting at fingertip down to the base. (See A below.)

    c. Halsted clamp the Penrose to itself at the base of the finger
       to secure it in place. (See B below.) (Fig. 7.6)

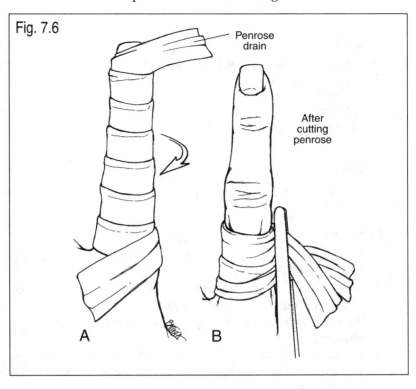

Fig. 7.6

Penrose drain

After cutting penrose

A   B

    d. Cut the Penrose distally along finger to expose the wound,
      leaving it and the Halsted intact at the base of the finger.

7. Complications and Management:

    a. Ischemia
      • Do not keep the tourniquet on for more than 1 hour.

B. ARM TOURNIQUET

1. Indications:

    Wounds of the forearm and hand

2. Contraindications:

    Previous surgery to the axilla

3. Anesthesia:

   Wrist block or field block

4. Equipment:

   a. Arm tourniquet or blood pressure cuff
   b. 1/2 inch cloth tape
   c. Soft roll cast padding
   d. Ace wrap
   e. Clamps

5. Positioning:

   Supine with arm extended on arm board

6. Technique:

   a. Place long piece of tape on volar aspect of arm and forearm longitudinally.
   b. Wrap 3–4 layers of cast padding around the arm at the level of the mid-humerus circumferentially.
   c. Place a tourniquet or blood pressure cuff around the cast padding.
   d. To secure the tourniquet's position, lift up distal end of tape, wrap it over the tourniquet, and tape distal end onto proximal end longitudinally.
   e. Hold the patient's hand over his head and exsanguinate the arm by tightly wrapping it with an Ace wrap, starting at the fingertips down to level of the tourniquet.
   f. Inflate the tourniquet to 100–150 mm Hg above patient's systolic pressure.
   g. Remove the Ace wrap.
   h. Clamp the tubing to the blood pressure cuff to prevent loss of pressure.

7. Complications and Management:

   a. Ischemia
      • Do not keep tourniquet on more than 1 hour.
      • The arm tourniquet is reasonably comfortable for 15 minutes alone and up to 1 hour when combined with a wrist block.

III. HAND PROCEDURES

A. REMOVAL OF A NAIL

1. Indications:
   a. Nailbed laceration
   b. Inadequately drained subungual hematoma
   c. Displaced tuft fractures
   d. Extensive paronychia
   e. Complex/crush injury of nail

2. Contraindications:
   None

3. Anesthesia:
   Digital block

4. Equipment:
   a. Sterile prep solution
   b. Sterile gloves and towels
   c. Halsted clamp
   d. Scissors

5. Positioning:
   Supine with the hand prone on an arm board

6. Technique:
   a. Sterile prep and drape finger and hand.
   b. Digital block as per section I.B.
   c. Without traumatizing the uninjured portions of the nailbed, carefully elevate nail from nailbed using a fine Halsted clamp (Fig. 7.7).
   d. Spread under the eponychium with the fine Halsted clamp to separate the nail from the eponychium. Cut the lateral edges of the eponychium with fine scissors, if necessary (Fig. 7.8).
   e. Once the nail is free from the nailbed on the deep surface and free from the eponychium on the superficial proximal surface, remove the nail by grasping the tip of the nail with the hemostat and gently pulling the nail straight out.

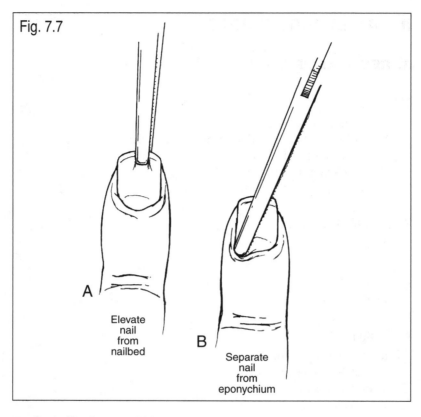

Fig. 7.7

A Elevate nail from nailbed

B Separate nail from eponychium

7. Complications and Management:

   a. Injury to nailbed: Repair as per section III.B.

B. REPAIR OF NAILBED LACERATION

1. Indications:

   Nailbed laceration

2. Contraindications:

   a. Displaced distal phalangeal tuft fracture (50% of all nailbed injuries)
   b. Must reduce tuft fracture prior to nailbed repair for normal healing.

3. Anesthesia:

   Digital block

Fig. 7.8

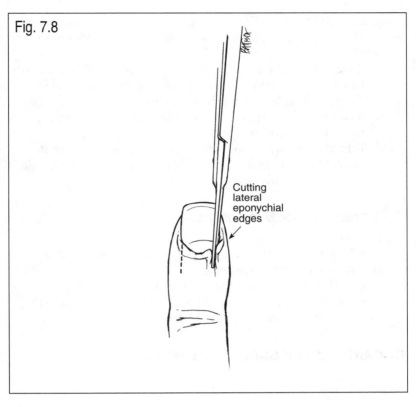

Cutting
lateral
eponychial
edges

4. Equipment:
   a. Sterile prep solution
   b. Sterile gloves and towels
   c. 30 mL syringe
   d. 19 gauge angio catheter
   e. Sterile saline
   f. Halsted clamp
   g. Scissors
   h. Needle driver
   i. 5–0 nylon suture
   j. 6–0 chromic suture on atraumatic needle

5. Positioning:
   Supine with arm extended on arm board and hand prone

6. Technique:
   a. Sterile prep and drape finger and hand.
   b. Remove nail as per section III.A.

c. Irrigate wound with sterile saline using 30 mL syringe with 19 gauge angio catheter. Use about 100 mL saline per inch of wound.

d. Repair the nailbed using simple interrupted 6–0 chromic sutures just deep enough to approximate the surface edges. Avoid hitting bone with deep stitches.

e. If eponychium or paronychia is cut, repair with simple interrupted 5–0 nylon suture.

f. Take the removed intact fingernail and place it under the eponychial fold in its normal anatomic position to provide splinting and protection.

7. Complications and Management:

a. Infection
  - May need to remove sutures and/or start soaks with saline to promote drainage.
  - Initiate antibiotics if there is surrounding cellulitis.
  - Elevate upper extremity and splint forearm/hand in the position of function. See Chapter 8.

C. DRAINAGE OF SUBUNGUAL HEMATOMA

1. Indications:

Subungual hematoma

2. Contraindications:

a. Distal phalangeal tuft fracture
b. Nailbed laceration

3. Anesthesia:

Digital block

4. Equipment:

a. Sterile prep solution
b. Sterile gloves and towels
c. Either a battery-operated cautery or 18 gauge needle

5. Positioning:

Supine with arm extended on arm board and hand prone

6. Technique:
    a. Sterile prep and drape finger and hand.
    b. If there is a nailbed laceration, distal tuft fracture, or if the nail is already broken/dislodged, remove nail as per section III.A.
    c. If no fracture, pierce the nail over hematoma collection just through the nail with the cautery or needle. Rotate back and forth to get through the nail when using a needle (Fig. 7.9).

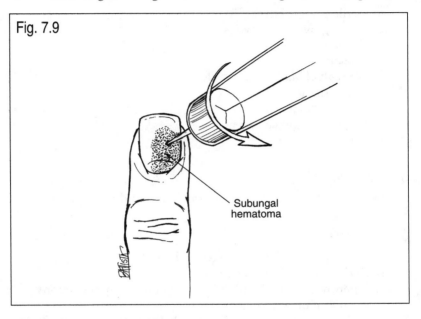

Fig. 7.9

Subungal hematoma

    d. If adequate drainage is achieved, old hematoma will easily escape through the hole as you press down on the nail around the hole.
    e. If adequate drainage is not achieved, remove the nail as per section III.A.

7. Complications and Management:
    a. Nailbed injury: Repair as per section III.B.

D. TREATMENT OF PARONYCHIA

1. Indications:

    Late paronychia (too large to be treated by soaks and antibiotics)

2. Contraindications:

None

3. Anesthesia:

Digital block

4. Equipment:

  a. Sterile prep solution
  b. Sterile gloves and towels
  c. Halsted clamp
  d. Scissors
  e. #15 scalpel blade and handle
  f. Sterile saline
  g. 30 mL syringe
  h. 19 gauge angio catheter
  i. Xeroform gauze

5. Positioning:

Supine with arm extended on arm board and hand prone

6. Technique:

  a. Sterile prep and drape finger and hand.
  b. Digital block as per section I.B.
  c. If paronychial fold and only small part of adjacent epony-
     chium involved,
     • Elevate only the lateral 1/3 nail closest to side of infection
       from nailbed with fine Halsted clamp (Fig. 7.10).
     • Cut nail longitudinally with fine scissors to isolate 1/3 of
       nail to be removed.
     • Free up 1/3 of eponychium from nail by spreading under
       eponychium with fine Halsted clamp.
     • Remove 1/3 of loosened nail.
  d. If infection is more extensive, remove entire nail as per sec-
     tion III.A.
  e. Incise eponychial fold to promote drainage if necessary.
  f. Irrigate wound with saline using a 30 mL syringe and 19
     gauge angio catheter.
  g. Dress wound with Xeroform to keep nailbed covered and
     skin edges open.
  h. Continue saline soaks.

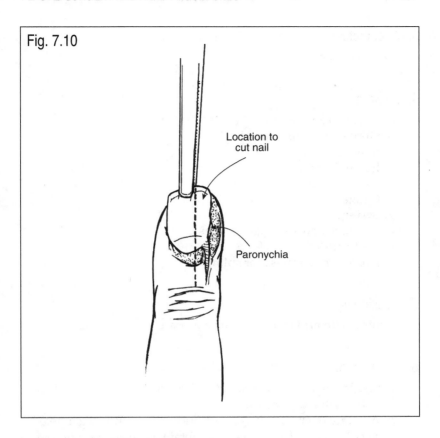

Fig. 7.10

Location to cut nail

Paronychia

7. Complications and Management:
   a. Inadequate drainage
      • Incise eponychial fold.
      • If still inadequate, remove nail per section III.A.
   b. Nailbed injury: Repair as per Section III.B.

E. INCISION AND DRAINAGE OF UPPER EXTREMITY ABSCESS

1. Indications:

   Superficial hand/forearm abscesses

2. Contraindications:
   a. Deep abscesses
   b. Abscess near important neurovascular structures

3. Anesthesia:

Local/field block

4. Equipment:

a. Sterile prep solution
b. Sterile gloves and towels
c. Scalpel
d. Halsted clamp
e. Sterile saline
f. Gauze
g. Syringe
h. 25 gauge and 18 gauge needles
i. Cast padding
j. Plaster or fiberglass for splint

5. Positioning:

Supine with arm extended on arm board

6. Technique:

a. Sterile prep and drape hand or forearm.
b. Administer anesthesia.
c. Aspirate over area of greatest fluctuation with 18 gauge needle to localize abscess and obtain a sample for microbiology.
d. Make an adequate incision over area of greatest fluctuation with scalpel. May need to make narrow elliptical incision to promote drainage.
e. Break up loculations with a Halsted clamp (Fig. 7.11).
f. Irrigate copiously with saline and pack the cavity with gauze.
g. Splint the forearm/hand in the position of function. See Chapter 8.

7. Complications and Management:

a. Inadequate drainage
  • Deep abscesses may require operative drainage.
b. Neurovascular injury
  • Observe.
  • May need operative repair.

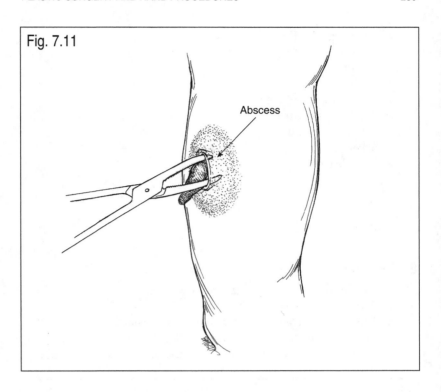

Fig. 7.11

Abscess

IV. COMPLEX LACERATIONS

A. LIP

1. Indications:

   Lip laceration

2. Contraindications:

   Laceration greater than 1/3 of lip length

3. Anesthesia:

   Local/field block

4. Equipment:

   a. Sterile prep solution
   b. Sterile gloves and towels

    c. 25 gauge needle
    d. 5 mL syringe
    e. Sterile saline
    f. Scalpel
    g. 4–0 chromic suture
    h. 4–0 Vicryl suture
    i. 6–0 nylon suture
    j. Scissors
    k. Needle driver

5. Positioning:

Supine

6. Technique:

    a. Sterile prep and drape lip and lower face.
    b. Administer local anesthesia.
    c. Trim edges of wound with scalpel or scissors if necessary and copiously irrigate wound with saline.
    d. If laceration is full-thickness, it must be closed in 3 layers:

Fig. 7.12

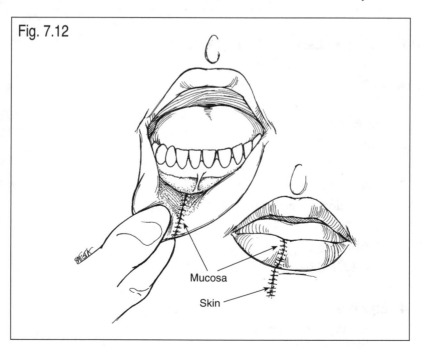

Mucosa

Skin

- Muscle: Approximate with 1 or 2 simple interrupted 4–0 Vicryl sutures.
- Mucosa: Approximate with simple interrupted 4–0 chromic sutures.
- Skin: Approximate edges with simple interrupted 6–0 nylon sutures, carefully aligning the skin-vermilion border.

B. EAR

1. Indications:

   Simple ear laceration

2. Contraindications:

   a. Grossly contaminated or human bite wounds should not be immediately closed.
   b. Amputated or near amputated ears require operative repair.

3. Anesthesia:

   Local/field block

4. Equipment:

   a. Sterile prep solution
   b. Sterile gloves and towels
   c. 25 gauge needle
   d. Syringe
   e. Needle driver
   f. Scissors, scalpel
   g. 5–0 nylon suture
   h. 4–0 Dexon suture
   i. Xeroform
   j. 4 × 4 gauze, fluffed gauze, 3-inch Kling gauze
   k. 3-inch Ace wrap

5. Positioning:

   Supine with head turned to one side

6. Technique:

   a. Sterile prep and drape ear.

   b. If the laceration involves skin and only a small cartilage defect, skin approximation is all that is needed to restore the auricular contour.

- Approximate the skin with simple interrupted 5–0 nylon sutures.
- If the laceration involves the rim of the ear, use a vertical mattress suture with 5–0 nylon along the rim to evert the edges, which will prevent a notched appearance at the rim (Fig. 7.13).

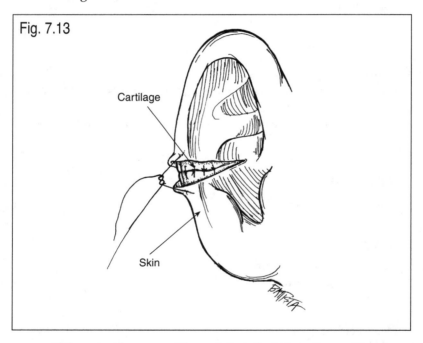

Fig. 7.13

Cartilage

Skin

   c. If there is a larger cartilage defect, first close the cartilage with simple interrupted 4–0 Dexon suture and tie the knots on the posterior side.

   d. If a hematoma is present below the skin of the external ear, drain the hematoma by making a small incision with the scalpel over the hematoma.

   e. Apply a compressive ear dressing.

- Pack Xeroform strips into ear crevices.
- Tuck a 4 × 4 gauze behind the ear.
- Place a wad of fluff gauze over ear.

- Wrap head and injured ear with a 3-inch Kling followed by a 3-inch Ace wrap, leaving the opposite ear free of dressing.

7. Complications and Management:
    a. Hematoma: Check wound in 24 hours. If a hematoma develops, it must be drained and a compressive dressing reapplied.
    b. Later complications include chondritis, stricture of external auditory canal, and keloid formation.

CHAPTER

ORTHOPEDIC PROCEDURES

Author: Jennifer M. Lindsey, M.D.

ORTHOPEDIC PROCEDURES

Musculoskeletal injuries are very commonly encountered by non-orthopedic medical practitioners. Many of these injuries can initially be managed before referral to the orthopedic surgeon. In this chapter, several general orthopedic techniques are described, including measurement of compartment pressures, arthrocentesis, splinting, and joint reductions.

A. MEASUREMENT OF COMPARTMENT PRESSURES

1. Indications:

Any condition where circulation and function of tissues within a closed space are compromised by an increase in compression within that space. Generally seen with forearm, lower leg, and rarely thigh injuries. Clinical signs include:
   a. Pain with passive motion (stretch) of tendon whose muscle originates in the compartment (first sign)
   b. Pain out of proportion to the injury and unrelenting
   c. Pallor
   d. Paresthesias (late sign)
   e. Paralysis (late sign)
   f. Pulselessness (late sign)
   If one waits for the appearance of these 6 P's, one will learn of an additional P—Plaintiff.

2. Contraindications:

   a. Coagulopathy
   b. Infection at site of puncture

3. Anesthesia:

None
a. Injection of local anesthetics can change intracompartmental pressure.
b. IV sedation prevents monitoring of clinical situation.

4. Equipment:

a. Stryker pressure and monitoring kit
b. Whiteside's technique
  • Sterile 20 mL Luer-Lock tip syringe
  • 4-way stopcock
  • Bottle of sterile saline
  • 35 inch extension tube sets (2)
  • 18 gauge needles (2)
  • Mercury manometer

5. Positioning:

Extremity to be measured is horizontal to ground and resting on flat surface.

6. Technique—Whiteside's Technique for Calf Pressures:

a. Assemble apparatus as shown with a 20 mL syringe spring set at 15 mL (Fig. 8.1).
b. Insert needle into bottle of sterile saline with stopcock closed to manometer.
c. Aspirate saline until half of the extension tube is filled.
d. Close stopcock to tubing with needle, then replace it with sterile 18 gauge needle.
e. Sterile prep and drape calf.
f. Insert 18 gauge needle into muscle of compartment to be measured.
  • Anterior compartment: muscle mass just lateral to the ridge of tibia
  • Lateral compartment: just anterior to fibula
  • Superficial posterior compartment: From medial aspect of calf, enter posterior muscle belly approximately 2–5 cm depending on patient's subcutaneous fat.
  • Deep posterior compartment: From position of superficial posterior compartment, angle anterior and advance needle into deep tissue.
g. Open stopcock to both extension tubes and syringe.

Fig. 8.1

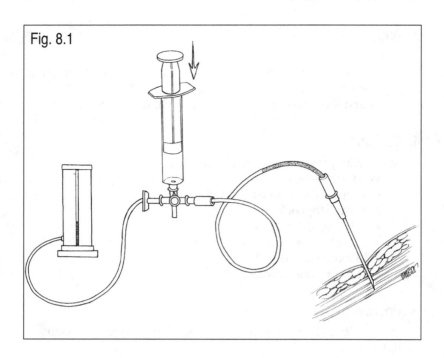

h. Slowly depress syringe plunger until air/saline meniscus moves.
i. When air/saline meniscus moves, read pressure on manometer and record.
j. Withdraw needle and enter next compartment to be measured.
k. When in doubt as to accuracy of readings, the uninjured contralateral extremity can be used as a control.
l. Technique can be modified for any compartment in the body.
m. Place sterile gauze over puncture site.
n. If pressure in compartment is more than 40 mm Hg, then open fasciotomy is indicated.

7. Complications and Management:
a. Error in reading if needle is against bone or in soft tissue
   • Double check each reading within the compartments.
   • Ensure that extremity and manometer are level.
   • Compare to opposite extremity.
   • If borderline, one should re-measure pressures one to two hours later.

   b. Infection at puncture sites
  - Local wound care
  - Oral or IV antibiotics

B. ARTHROCENTESIS

1. Indications:
   a. Post-traumatic hemarthrosis
   b. Joint fluid analysis
   c. Intraarticular injections
   d. Septic arthritis

2. Contraindications:
   a. Overlying cellulitis
   b. Coagulopathy (especially hemophilia)

3. Anesthesia:
   1% lidocaine subcutaneously

4. Equipment:
   a. Sterile prep set
   b. Sterile gloves and drapes
   c. 18 gauge needle
   d. 20 mL syringes (2)
   e. Small Kelly clamp
   f. One lavender (EDTA) top and one green (Heparinized) top sample tube
   g. Culture swabs
   h. 5 mL syringe
   j. 25 gauge needle
   k. 1% lidocaine

5. Positioning:
   a. Knee/ankle: Rest knee or ankle on stretcher.
   b. Shoulder: Patient is seated with affected arm hanging off stretcher.
   c. Elbow: Rest elbow on table in flex position with forearm pronated.
   d. Wrist: Rest wrist on table with hand pronated.

6. Approaches:

    a. Ankle: Insert needle 2.5 cm proximal and 1.3 cm medial to the tip of the lateral malleolus (Fig. 8.2).

Fig. 8.2

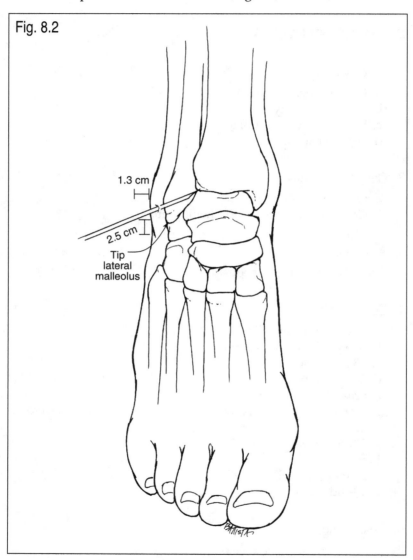

    b. Knee: Insert needle laterally at level of superior pole of patella then advance into the joint (Fig. 8.3).
    c. Shoulder: Insert needle at one-half the distance between the coracoid process and anterolateral edge of the

Fig. 8.3

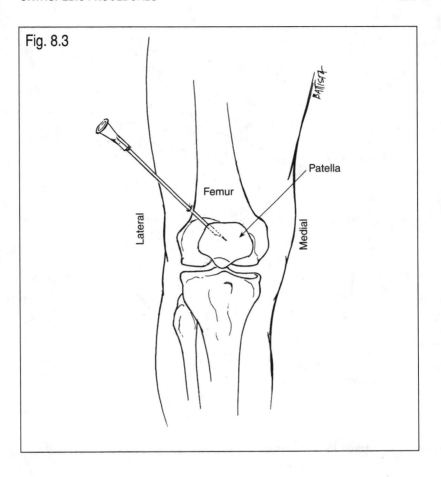

acromion. Direct needle posteriorly and enter joint. May
need to rotate arm internally and externally to find entrance point (Fig. 8.4).
d. Elbow: Insert needle at posterior aspect just lateral to the
olecranon (Fig. 8.5).
e. Wrist: Insert needle at base of snuff box just adjacent to the
extensor pollicis longus (EPL). Snuff box is palpable when
patient abducts thumb. EPL tendon palpable when patient
extends and flexes index finger (Fig. 8.6).

7. Technique:
   a. Sterile prep and drape entire joint.
   b. At site of approach, inject 1% lidocaine subcutaneously to
      raise a wheal with a 25 gauge needle.

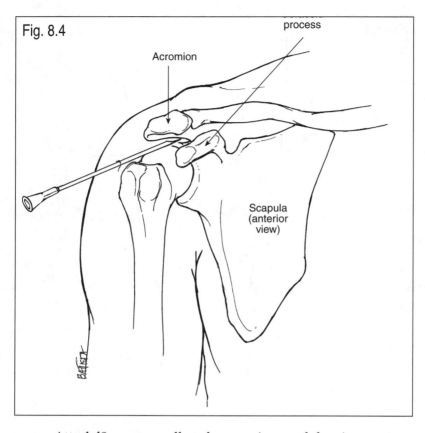

Fig. 8.4

Coracoid process

Acromion

Scapula (anterior view)

c. Attach 18 gauge needle to large syringe and then insert at site of anesthesia into the joint.
d. Aspirate fluid from the joint. May need to use other hand to milk fluid from recesses in joint into the area where the needle is located.
e. If the entire syringe is filled, use a small clamp to hold the needle in position and then change to a new syringe.
f. When all the fluid is aspirated, withdraw needle and dress with sterile gauze.
g. Splint joint in position of function. (See Section C.)
h. Send fluid for the following studies:
   • Lavender tube: cell count and differential
   • Green tube: crystal analysis
   • Culture swabs: culture and sensitivity, gram stain

8. Complications and Management:

a. Superficial infection at puncture site

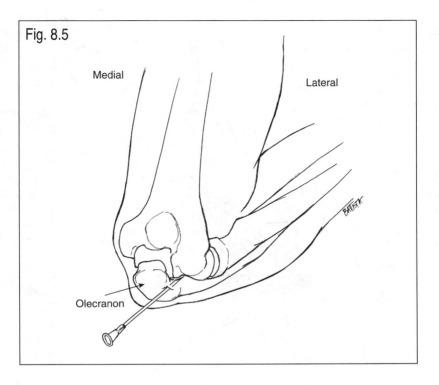

Fig. 8.5

Medial

Lateral

Olecranon

- Local wound care
- Oral or IV antibiotics
b. Deep infection
  - Joint seeded with bacteria when needle passed through cellulitis or inadequate sterile technique.
  - IV antibiotics
  - Open irrigation and débridement of joint
c. Bleeding
  - Compression dressing
  - Treat coagulopathy if present.

C. SPLINTING

1. Indications:
   a. Fracture
   b. Dislocated joint after reduction
   c. Sprain: torn or stretched ligaments
   d. Strain: torn or stretched muscles or tendons
   e. Post-operative immobilization

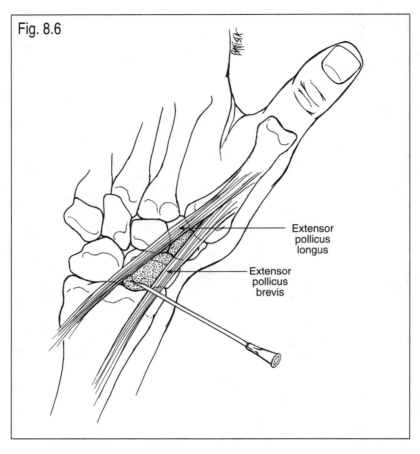

Fig. 8.6

Extensor pollicus longus

Extensor pollicus brevis

2. Contraindications:
   a. Absolute: none
   b. Relative: Injuries involving open wounds or infections need easily removable splints to allow soft tissue care.

3. Anesthesia:
   If injury is grossly stable, use IV sedation. (See Appendix B.)

4. Equipment:
   a. Cast padding (soft roll)
   b. Plaster/fiberglass
   c. Lukewarm water
   d. Ace bandages
   e. Disposable gloves

5. Positioning:

a. Ankle/foot: 90° angle between foot and leg, neutral eversion/inversion
b. Knee: 15–20° flexion
c. Shoulder: resting at the side of the body
d. Elbow: 90° angle between forearm and arm, neutral pronation/supination
e. Wrist: neutral supination/pronation, 20–30° wrist extension
f. Thumb: wrist position as above, thumb in 45° abduction, 30° flexion
g. Metacarpals, MCP joint, proximal phalanges: wrist position as above, MCP joint in 90° flexion, DIP and PIP joint in full extension
h. IP joints, middle/distal phalanx: full extension at IP joints

6. Technique:

a. Splint padding
   - Apply soft roll to entire area to be splinted with 2–3" proximal and distal overhang.
   - Padding should be applied evenly in a circular fashion from distal to proximal with each turn overlapping by 50% of the next turn to allow at least two layers of soft roll in all areas.
   - Apply extra layers to bony prominences.
   - Apply soft roll while limb is in final splint position to prevent bunching of padding across joint flexion creases.
b. Fiberglass/plaster
   - General technique: immobilize fracture one joint above and one joint below injury.
   - Prefabricated fiberglass splints can be measured and cut.
   - Plaster splints need 10–12 layers of plaster in upper extremities and 12–15 layers of plaster in lower extremities.
   - Splints are dipped in room temperature or lukewarm water.
   - Excess water is gently squeezed or shaken from the splint.
   - Splint is applied to the soft roll and never directly onto the skin. The splint is held in place by an assistant or the patient.
c. Ace wrap
   - Wrap Ace bandage around splint with gentle tension.
   - Ace wrap should never be tight enough to cause venous compression.

Fig. 8.7

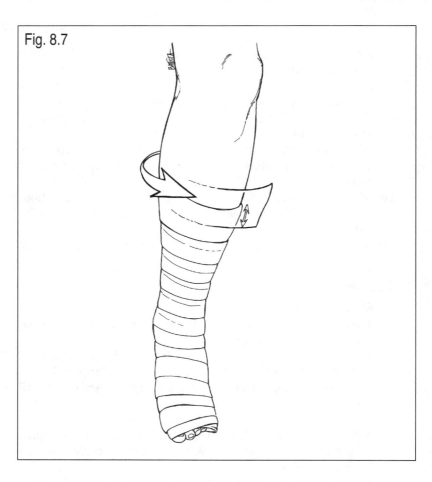

- Hold extremity in desired position until splint hardens (approximately 5–10 minutes with fiberglass, 10–15 minutes with plaster).

7. Specific Splints:
   a. Posterior elbow splint (Fig. 8.8)
      - Begin 4″ wide splint from posterior upper arm across the posterior elbow.
      - Extend the splint over the ulnar border of the forearm and hand to just proximal to the MCP joint.
   b. Sugar tong forearm splint (Fig. 8.9)
      - Use for forearm/wrist injuries.
      - Begin with 3–4″ wide splint in the palm of the hand at the level of the MCP joints.

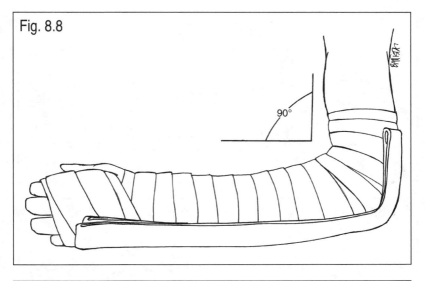

Fig. 8.8

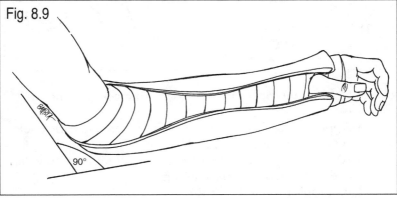

Fig. 8.9

- Extend splint up dorsal aspect of the forearm, around the elbow flexed at 90°, down the volar aspect of the forearm and hand, to just proximal to the MCP joint.
- Be sure that the splint does not limit MCP motion.
c. Ulnar gutter splint (Fig. 8.10)
- Used for fourth and fifth metacarpal or phalanx injuries.
- Apply 3–4" wide slab from ulnar aspect of proximal forearm down along the ulnar aspect of the small finger.
- Fold edges around dorsal and volar aspect of hand and ring/small fingers.
- Place the wrist in neutral supination/pronation with 20–30° extension.
d. Radial gutter splint (Fig. 8.11)

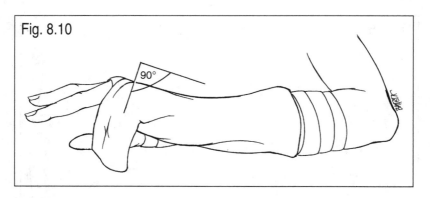

Fig. 8.10

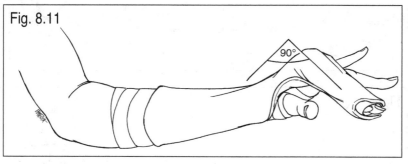

Fig. 8.11

- Used for injuries of the second/third metacarpal or fingers.
- Apply to radial border as above for ulnar side with a hole cut out to allow motion of the thumb.
- Alternatively, apply two separate 2–3″ wide slabs to volar and dorsal aspect of hand and fingers.

e. Thumb spica splint (Fig. 8.12)

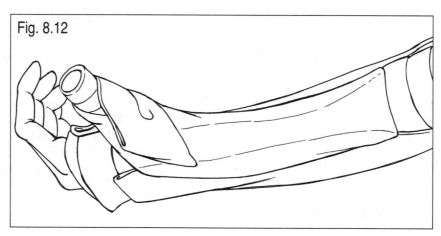

Fig. 8.12

- Apply Sugar tong splint as above.
- Add an additional 3" wide slab from upper forearm, along radial border, then down around thumb.
- Thumb IP joint should be included.

f. Long leg splint (Fig. 8.13)

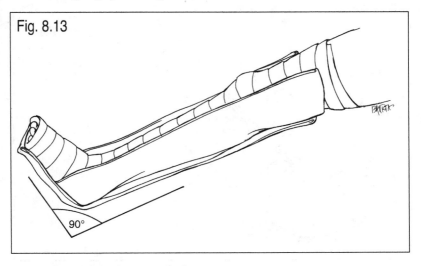

Fig. 8.13

90°

- Used for knee and tibia injuries.
- Apply 4" wide splint beginning at the medial upper thigh extending down the medial knee and ankle.
- Continue the splint around the heel and up the lateral side of the ankle and knee to the lateral upper thigh.
- This should form a U shape.
- For additional stability, apply a 6" splint from the posterior upper thigh down the posterior aspect of the leg and plantar surface of the foot.

g. Ankle splint (Fig. 8.14)

- Use for isolated ankle injuries.
- Apply 4" wide splint beginning at the proximal border of the upper calf extending down the medial calf and ankle around the heel and up the lateral ankle and lateral calf.
- For additional stability apply a 6" splint from the posterior upper calf down the posterior aspect of the lower leg and the plantar surface of the foot.

8. Complications and Management:

a. Burns
- Splints harden by exothermic reaction and can burn underlying skin.

Fig. 8.14

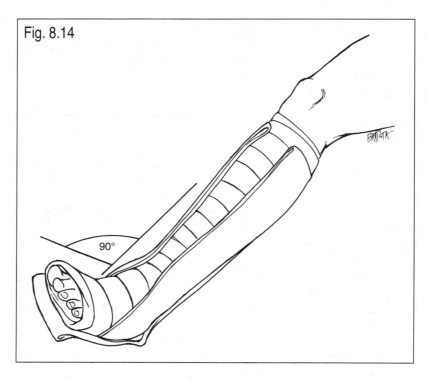

- Be sure skin is properly padded.
- Never use hot water to moisten splints.
- Avoid overly thick splints.
- If patient complains of significant heat or pain, remove splint and check the underlying skin.
- If burn occurs, treat with local burn techniques including débridement if necessary and topical Silvadene.

b. Cast sores
- Compression of skin over extended periods can lead to necrosis and breakdown.
- Be sure all bony and tendinous prominences are well padded.
- Be cautious about applying splints in unconscious patients or patients with insensate skin.
- If patient complains of burning pain or discomfort, remove splint and inspect skin.
- If splint is foul-smelling or drainage appears, remove splint immediately and inspect.
- If wound develops, treat with local wound care.
- Avoid indenting the splint with finger pressure while it is hardening.

   c. Joint contracture
- Long-term immobilization can lead to shortening of ligaments and tendons if improperly positioned.
- Check and re-check position of splint as it hardens.
- Avoid immobilization for longer than three weeks for shoulders and elbow injuries; six to eight weeks for any other injury.
- If contracture develops, begin physical therapy immediately.
- Orthopedics consult

D. CLOSED JOINT REDUCTION

1. Indications:
   a. Clinically or radiographically dislocated joint.

2. Contraindications:
   a. Shoulder dislocation: humeral shaft fracture
   b. Radial head dislocation: radial shaft fracture
   c. Ankle dislocation: tibial shaft fracture

3. Anesthesia:
   IV sedation (See Appendix B.)

4. Equipment:
   a. Shoulder: shoulder immobilizer
   b. Elbow: sling
   c. Ankle:
- Cast padding (soft roll)
- Plaster/fiberglass
- Lukewarm water
- Ace bandages
- Disposable gloves

5. Positioning:
   a. Shoulder
- Patient is resting on stretcher supine with the head of the bed at 30°.
- Stretcher should be at waist level of the person performing reduction.

- Patient's injured arm should be placed at the edge of the bed.
b. Radial head dislocation
    - Patient is seated comfortably with the hand of the injured extremity resting in the patient's lap.
c. Ankle
    - Patient seated on stretcher with legs dangling over the edge of the bed.

6. Technique:

a. Shoulder (Fig. 8.15)

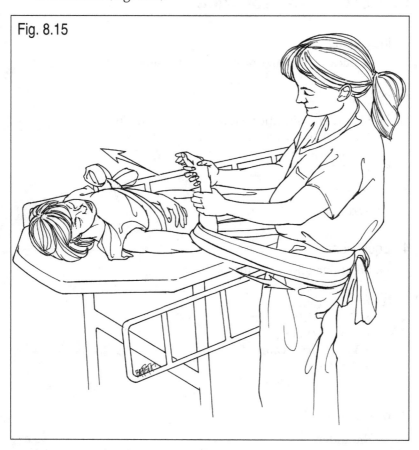

Fig. 8.15

- Wrap sheet around patient's trunk and tie to the opposite side of the bed rails.
- Tie a second sheet loosely around your waist (person performing the procedure).

- Place the forearm of the injured extremity into the sheet around your waist with the elbow flexed at 90°.
- Gently lean your body-weight backwards to create longitudinal traction on patient's arm abducted at 30° and internally rotated 15–30° for an anterior shoulder dislocation (rotation is external if shoulder is posteriorly dislocated).
- Hold traction for several minutes to fatigue shoulder girdle musculature.
- Gently externally rotate and abduct arm for anterior dislocation. For posterior dislocation, rotate the arm internally.
- May need to add additional pressure to humeral head with the hand.
- Shoulder should "click" back into position.
- If unsure about reduction, stop, and repeat radiographs.
- Always check post-reduction radiographs (AP and Y views) to confirm and document adequate position.
- Place the arm in shoulder immobilizer.

b. Radial head (Fig. 8.16)

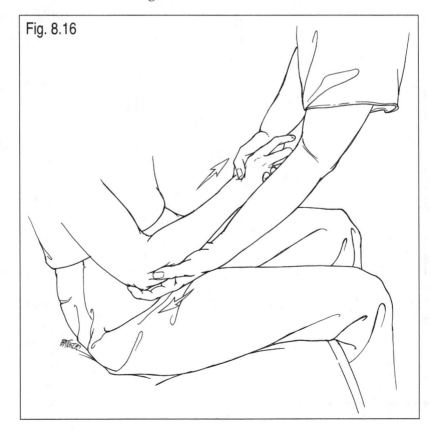

Fig. 8.16

- Grasp hand of injured extremity in the handshake position.
- Place the other hand behind the elbow with the thumb on the radial head.
- Gently pull longitudinal traction.
- Supinate forearm while keeping pressure on the radial head with the thumb.
- If needed, hyperflex elbow while keeping pressure on the radial head.
- Always check post-reduction radiographs (AP and lateral views) to confirm and document adequate position.
- Place the arm in a sling.

c. Ankle (Fig. 8.17)

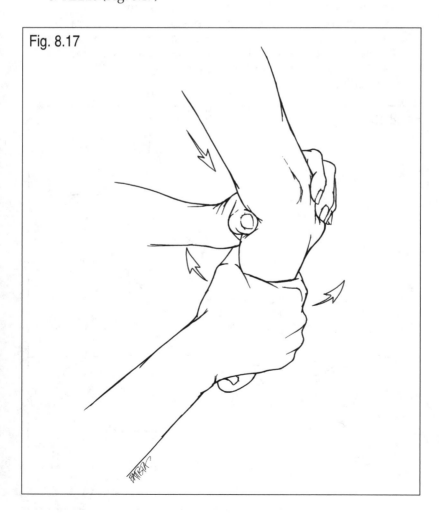

Fig. 8.17

- Have an assistant stabilize the legs by placing pressure on the patient's thighs.
- Grasp the forefoot with one hand and the heel with your other hand.
- Re-create mechanism of injury by twisting the foot towards the side that the talus is dislocated.
- Apply longitudinal traction.
- Reverse mechanism of injury to pull talus back under the tibia.
- Always check post-reduction radiographs (AP, lateral, mortis views) to confirm and document adequate position.
- Splint as in section C.

7. Complications and Management:

a. Fracture
  - Splint as needed.
  - Orthopedics consult
b. Unable to reduce dislocation
  - Splint and immobilize in position that is most comfortable for patient.
  - Orthopedic consult

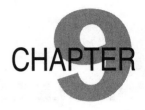

CHAPTER 9

NEEDLE BIOPSIES

Author: Attila Nakeeb, M.D.

NEEDLE BIOPSIES

Needle biopsies have been used to differentiate benign and malignant lesions since the late 1800s. It has become a powerful clinical tool for the evaluation of both palpable and nonpalpable lesions. For surgeons, needle biopsy of palpable lesions can be an efficient, simple, and safe technique for obtaining a tissue diagnosis in the outpatient setting or at the bedside.

Bedside needle biopsies can be subdivided into two types: (1) fine needle aspiration (FNA) biopsy, in which a small gauge needle is used to obtain a sample of cells for cytologic evaluation and (2) large needle cutting biopsy (LNCB), in which a trocar and large bore needle are used to obtain a cylinder of tissue for histologic evaluation. These techniques have been used extensively for the evaluation of lesions of the head and neck, thyroid, breast, liver, kidney, and soft tissue.

I. FINE NEEDLE ASPIRATION (FNA)

A. THYROID

1. Indications:

   a. Evaluation of palpable thyroid masses
   b. Differentiation of benign from malignant thyroid lesions

2. Contraindications:

   None

3. Anesthesia:

Anesthesia is not routinely used for FNA. However, if needed, a small amount of 1% lidocaine can be infiltrated locally, taking care not to distort the palpable lesion.

4. Equipment:

   a. Alcohol prep
   b. 10 mL syringe
   c. 1/2-inch 25 gauge needle
   d. Syringe holder (optional)
   e. Glass microscope slides (2)
   f. Spray fixative, gauze
   g. In many situations, it may be preferable to have a cy-
      topathologist present.

5. Positioning:

The patient is placed in a supine position and a roll is placed behind the shoulders to allow for neck extension and to bring the lesion closer to the surface (Fig. 9.1).

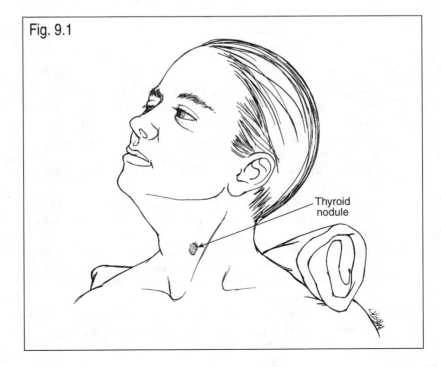

Fig. 9.1

Thyroid nodule

6. Technique:

    a. Prep the area for aspiration with an alcohol prep pad as if for phlebotomy.

    b. Palpate the lesion and immobilize the mass between the fingertips of the nondominant hand (Fig. 9.2).

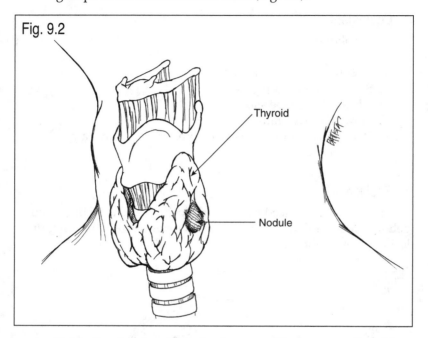

Fig. 9.2

Thyroid

Nodule

    c. Using the dominant hand, advance a 25 gauge needle with an attached 10 mL syringe into the lesion. The needle should be directed medially, towards the trachea (Fig. 9.3).

    d. Note the consistency of the mass upon entering it with the needle (firm, soft, rubbery, doughy, gritty).

    e. *Once the lesion is entered,* a full 10 mL of suction is applied to the syringe.

    f. While maintaining suction, move the needle back and forth through the lesion several times in different directions (Fig. 9.4).

    g. Release the syringe plunger and allow it to return to a neutral position prior to removing the needle from the lesion. At this point the specimen is within the needle and hub and should not be in the syringe.

    h. Remove the needle from the patient and have the patient apply pressure to the puncture site with a gauze pad.

    i. Detach the needle from the syringe.

    j. Fill the syringe with air.

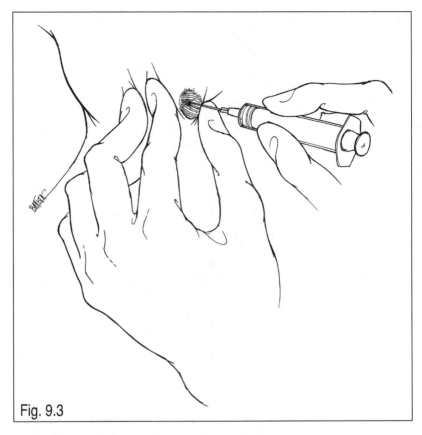

Fig. 9.3

   k. Reattach the needle onto the syringe.
   l. Touch the needle tip to a glass microscope slide with the
      bevel at a 45–90° angle to the slide surface.
  m. Expel material within the needle onto the slide.
   n. Make a smear by using a second glass slide to gently press
      down and draw out the material to a feathered edge. If the
      material is more liquid, it is pulled in the same fashion as a
      blood smear, except that before the feathering process is
      completed, the spreading slide is raised leaving a line of
      particles across the slide. The spreading slide is then turned
      and again pressed down against the line of particles and
      drawn out into a feathered edge.
   o. Air dry or apply cytological fixative to the slide as per the
      protocol of the cytopathology laboratory that will be process-
      ing the specimen. (If a fixative is applied it must be applied
      very quickly, usually within seconds of preparing the smear.)
   p. Most cytopathologists require 3–6 needle passes (samples)
      for an adequate pathologic diagnosis.

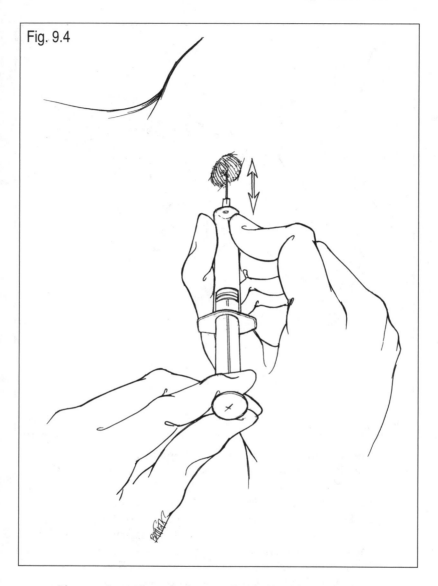

Fig. 9.4

q. If a cyst is aspirated, the cyst fluid should be sent for cytology. The region of the cyst should then be reexamined; if a residual mass is felt, it should then undergo FNA.

7. Complications and Management:

a. Bleeding and hematomas
- Thyroid punctures may produce significant hematomas and ecchymoses.

- Apply firm direct pressure to puncture sites immediately following aspiration.
  b. Tracheal puncture
     - If the trachea is entered, the suction in the syringe will be lost, and the aspiration will need to be repeated.
     - Puncture is usually of no consequence due to small gauge of the needle.
  c. Infection
     - Extremely rare in FNA
     - Antibiotics as appropriate
     - Incision and drainage as necessary

B. BREAST, LYMPH NODE, AND SOFT TISSUE

1. Indications:

a. Evaluation of palpable masses
b. Aspiration of breast cysts
c. Differentiation of benign from malignant lesions

2. Contraindications:

None

3. Anesthesia:

Anesthesia is not routinely used for FNA. However, if needed, a small amount of 1% lidocaine can be infiltrated locally taking care not to distort the palpable lesion.

4. Equipment:

a. Alcohol prep
b. 10 mL syringe
c. 1 1/2-inch 25 gauge needle
d. Syringe holder (optional)
e. Glass microscope slides (2)
f. Spray fixative
g. Gauze

5. Positioning:

a. Breast: For upper quadrant lesions the patient is placed in an upright seated position. Lower quadrant lesions are better managed in a supine position.
b. Lymph node and soft tissue: depends on location of lesion

6. Technique:

a. Prep the area for aspiration with an alcohol prep pad as if for phlebotomy.

b. Palpate the lesion and immobilize the mass between the fingertips of the nondominant hand.

c. Using the dominant hand, advance a 25 gauge needle with an attached 10 mL syringe into the lesion (Fig. 9.5).

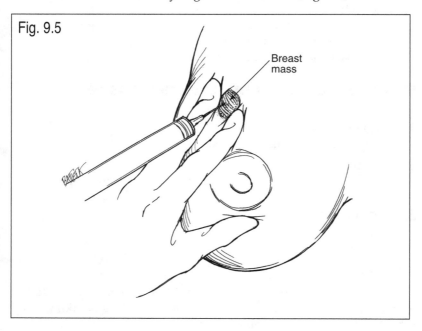

Fig. 9.5

Breast mass

d. Note the consistency of the mass upon entering it with the needle (firm, soft, rubbery, doughy, gritty).

e. *Once the lesion is entered,* a full 10 mL of suction is applied to the syringe.

f. While maintaining suction, move the needle back and forth through the lesion several times in different directions (Fig. 9.6).

g. Release the syringe plunger and allow it to return to a neutral position prior to removing the needle from the lesion. At this point the specimen is within the needle and hub and should not be in the syringe.

h. Remove the needle from the patient and have the patient apply pressure to the puncture site with a gauze pad.

i. Detach the needle from the syringe.

j. Fill the syringe with air.

Fig. 9.6

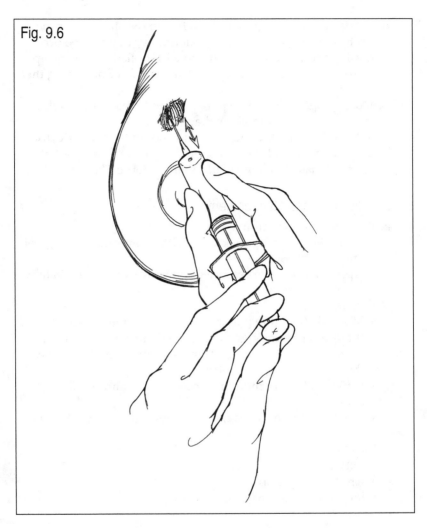

k. Reattach the needle onto the syringe.
l. Touch the needle tip to a glass microscope slide with the bevel at a 45–90° angle to the slide surface.
m. Expel material within the needle onto the slide.
n. Make a smear by using a second glass slide to gently press down and draw out the material to a feathered edge. If the material is more liquid, it is pulled in the same fashion as a blood smear, except that before the feathering process is completed, the spreading slide is raised leaving a line of particles across the slide. The spreading slide is then turned and again pressed down against the line of particles and drawn out into a feathered edge.

o. Air dry or apply cytological fixative to the slide as per the protocol of the cytopathology laboratory that will be processing the specimen. (If a fixative is applied it must be applied very quickly, usually within seconds of preparing the smear.)

p. Most cytopathologists require 3–6 needle passes (samples) for an adequate pathologic diagnosis.

q. If a cyst is aspirated, the cyst fluid should be sent for cytology. The region of the cyst should then be reexamined; if a residual mass is felt, it should then undergo FNA.

8. Complications and Management:

a. Bleeding and hematomas
- Breast FNA can be associated with significant hematomas and ecchymoses.
- Apply firm direct pressure to puncture sites immediately following aspiration.

b. Pneumothorax
- More likely in thin patients and deep lesions
- If tension pneumothorax suspected, decompression with 16 gauge IV into second intercostal space and then tube thoracostomy (see Chapter 3).
- If 10 to 20% pneumothorax, observation and serial chest X-rays.
- If >20% pneumothorax, tube thoracostomy per Chapter 3.

c. Infection
- Extremely rare in FNA
- Antibiotics as appropriate
- Incision and drainage as necessary

II. LARGE NEEDLE CUTTING BIOPSIES

A. SILVERMAN NEEDLE BIOPSY (SOFT TISSUE)

1. Indications:

a. To differentiate benign and malignant lesions

2. Contraindications:

a. Coagulopathy (PT or PTT >1.3 ratio, or platelets <20,000).

3. Anesthesia:

1% lidocaine locally

4. Equipment:

a. Sterile prep solution
b. Sterile gloves and towels
c. 5 mL syringe
d. 22 and 25 gauge needles
e. Scalpel blade
f. Silverman needle (Fig. 9.7)

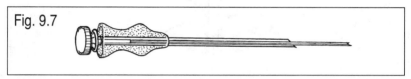

Fig. 9.7

g. Sterile dressing

5. Positioning:

The best patient position is when the lesion can be easily pal-pated and fixed into place by the examiner using one hand. For most biopsies the supine position is preferred. In thyroid and neck aspirations a roll is placed behind the shoulders which allows for neck extension and brings the lesion closer to the surface.

6. Technique:

a. Sterile prep and drape the lesion to be biopsied.
b. Infiltrate the skin overlying the 1% lidocaine using a 25 gauge needle.
c. Using the 22 gauge needle, infiltrate the subcutaneous tissue down to the mass with anesthetic.
d. Make a 5 mm incision in the skin and subcutaneous tissue with a scalpel.
e. Insert the Silverman needle with the obturator in place into the skin incision to the edge of the mass.
f. Remove the obturator and place cutting insert into the outer sheath and advance into the mass (Fig. 9.8).
g. Advance the outer sheath by rotation over the cutting insert to the tip. This maneuver severs the specimen within the blades of the cutting insert (Fig. 9.9).
h. Remove the needle with the outer sheath advanced over the

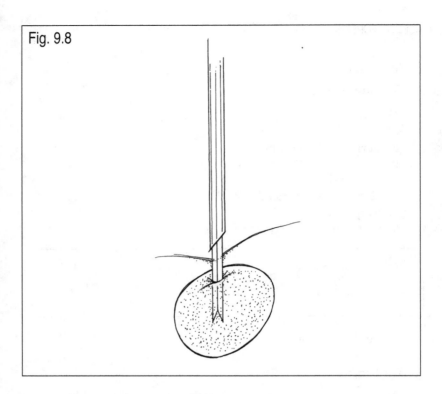

Fig. 9.8

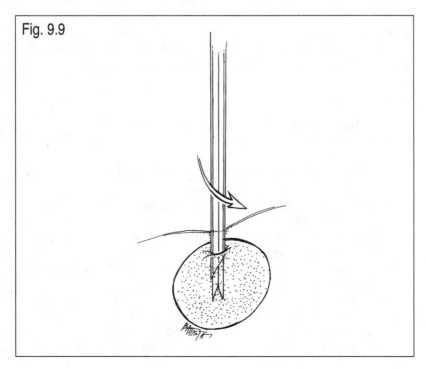

Fig. 9.9

cutting insert. Retrieve the specimen and send to pathology for processing.

i. Apply a clean sterile dressing to wound and apply pressure for 20–30 minutes.

7. Complications and Management:

a. Bleeding and hematomas
- Apply firm direct pressure to puncture sites immediately following aspiration.
- Correct coagulation abnormalities.

b. Infection
- Antibiotics as appropriate
- Incision and drainage as necessary

B. TRU-CUT NEEDLE BIOPSY (SOFT TISSUE)

1. Indications:

a. To differentiate benign and malignant lesions

2. Contraindications:

a. Coagulopathy (PT or PTT >1.3 ratio, or platelets <20,000).

3. Anesthesia:

1% lidocaine locally

4. Equipment:

a. Sterile prep solution
b. Sterile gloves and towels
c. 5 mL syringe
d. 22 and 25 gauge needles
e. Scalpel blade
f. Tru-cut needle (Fig. 9.10)

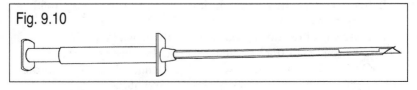

Fig. 9.10

g. Sterile dressings

5. Positioning:

The best patient position is when the lesion can be easily palpated and fixed into place by the examiner using one hand. For most biopsies the supine position is preferred. In thyroid and neck aspirations a roll is placed behind the shoulders which allows for neck extension and brings the lesion closer to the surface.

6. Technique:

    a. Sterile prep and drape the lesion to be biopsied.

    b. Infiltrate the skin overlying the 1% lidocaine using a 25 gauge needle.

    c. Using the 22 gauge needle, infiltrate the subcutaneous tissue down to the mass with anesthetic.

    d. Make a 5 mm incision in the skin and subcutaneous tissue with a scalpel.

    e. Fully retract the obturator of the Tru-Cut needle so that the specimen notch is covered (Fig. 9.11).

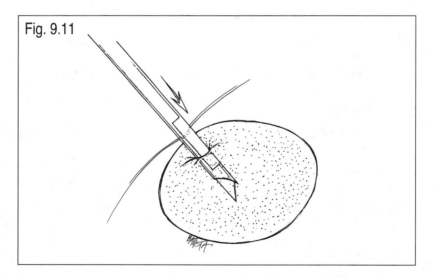

Fig. 9.11

    f. Insert the needle into the lesion so that the specimen notch is within the lesion to be biopsied (Fig. 9.12).

    g. Hold the obturator in place and pull outward on the T-shaped cannula handle to expose the specimen notch.

    h. Quickly but carefully advance the T-shaped cannula handle over the obturator to sever the tissue that had prolapsed into the open specimen notch (Fig. 9.13).

Fig. 9.12

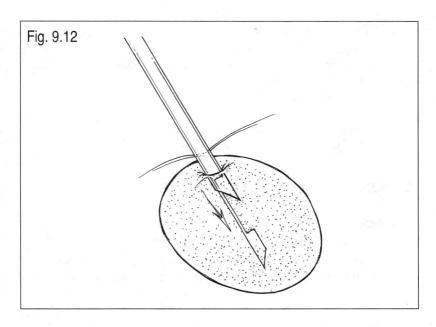

Fig. 9.13

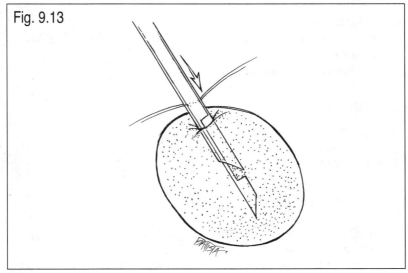

i. Remove the Tru-Cut needle with the cannula in the advanced position over the obturator.

j. Advance the obturator to expose the specimen notch and remove the tissue for pathology.

k. Apply a clean sterile dressing to wound and apply pressure for 20–30 minutes.

7. Complications and Management:

   a. Bleeding and hematomas
- Apply firm direct pressure to puncture sites immediately following aspiration.
- Correct coagulation abnormalities.

   b. Infection
- Antibiotics as appropriate
- Incision and drainage as necessary

C. PERCUTANEOUS LIVER BIOPSY

1. Indications:

   a. Diagnosis of primary liver disease
   b. Assessment of the progression of chronic liver disease
   c. Detection of malignant primary or metastatic disease
   d. Documentation of rejection in liver transplant patients

2. Contraindications:

   a. Uncooperative patient
   b. Coagulopathy (PT or PTT >1.3 ratio, or platelets <20,000)
   c. Local infection
   d. Massive tense ascites

3. Anesthesia:

   1% lidocaine locally

4. Equipment:

   a. Sterile prep solution
   b. Sterile gloves and towels
   c. 5 mL syringe
   d. 22 and 25 gauge needles
   e. Scalpel blade
   f. Tru-cut biopsy needle
   g. Sterile dressing

5. Positioning:

   Percutaneous liver biopsy is performed with the patient in the supine position with the patient's right arm tucked behind the head. Warn the patient of the possibility of sharp pain with radiation to the right shoulder.

6. Technique:

    a. Map the liver by percussion (or ultrasound). Mark the
      biopsy site on the skin 2–3 cm above the caudal margin of
      the liver in the midaxillary line.

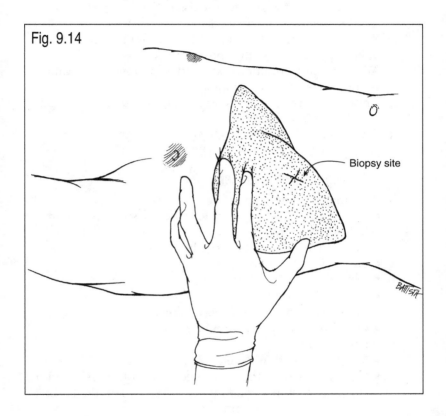

Fig. 9.14

Biopsy site

    b. Sterile prep and drape the right upper quadrant of the ab-
      domen.
    c. Infiltrate the skin with 1% lidocaine over the biopsy
      site.
    d. Using a 22 gauge needle, infiltrate the subcutaneous tissue
      with local anesthetic. With a scalpel blade, make a 5 mm
      skin incision.
    e. Fully retract the obturator of the Tru-Cut needle so that the
      specimen notch is covered.
    f. Ask the patient to take a deep breath and hold it.
    g. Insert the needle into the liver so that the specimen notch is
      within the lesion to be biopsied. The needle should only
      need to be inserted 2–4 cm.

h. Ask the patient to exhale and hold their breath.
i. Hold the obturator in place and pull outward on the T-shaped cannula handle to expose the specimen notch.
j. Quickly but carefully advance the T-shaped cannula handle over the obturator to sever the tissue that had prolapsed into the open specimen notch.
k. Remove the Tru-Cut needle with the cannula in the advanced position over the obturator.
l. Advance the obturator to expose the specimen notch and remove the tissue for pathology.
m. Apply a clean sterile dressing to wound and apply pressure for 20–30 minutes.
n. Patient should lie on the right side for at least two hours.

7. Complications and Management:
   a. Bleeding and hematoma
      • Apply firm direct pressure to puncture sites immediately following aspiration.
      • Correct coagulation abnormalities.
      • Surgical exploration if necessary
   b. Infection
      • Antibiotics as appropriate
      • Incision and drainage as necessary
      • Operative drainage as necessary
   c. Pneumothorax
      • More likely in thin patients and deep lesions
      • If tension pneumothorax suspected, decompression with 16 gauge IV into second intercostal space and then tube thoracostomy (see Chapter 3).
      • If 10–20% pneumothorax, observation and serial chest X-rays.
      • If >20% pneumothorax, tube thoracostomy per Chapter 3.

D. PERCUTANEOUS KIDNEY BIOPSY

1. Indications:
   a. Diagnosis of primary renal disease
   b. Assessment of the progression of chronic renal disease
   c. Documentation of rejection in renal transplant patients

2. Contraindications:

   a. Uncooperative patient
   b. Coagulopathy (PT or PTT >1.3 ratio, or platelets <30,000)
   c. Severe uncontrolled hypertension
   d. Known or suspected renal parenchymal infection
   e. Solitary ectopic or horseshoe kidney (except renal transplant)

3. Anesthesia:

   1% lidocaine locally

4. Equipment:

   a. Sterile prep solution
   b. Sterile gloves and towels
   c. 5 mL syringe
   d. 22 and 25 gauge needles
   e. Scalpel blade
   f. Biopsy needle (Silverman needle or Tru-cut needle)
   g. Sterile dressing
   h. Ultrasound
   i. Locating needle (22 gauge spinal needle)

5. Positioning:

   Percutaneous renal biopsy is performed with the patient in the prone position with a roll placed under the patient between the rib cage and the pelvis. Transplant biopsies are performed with the patient in a supine position.

6. Technique:

   a. Sterile prep and drape the appropriate flank area.
   b. Confirm the position of the kidney by ultrasound. Using a 25 gauge needle, infiltrate the skin with 1% lidocaine over the biopsy site (lower pole of kidney).
   c. Using a 22 gauge needle, infiltrate the subcutaneous tissue with local anesthetic.
   d. Make a 5 mm incision through the skin and subcutaneous tissue with a scalpel blade.
   e. Ask the patient to hold his or her breath in inspiration and

advance the locating needle is under ultrasound guidance into the kidney.

f. Release the needle and ask the patient to breathe in and out normally. If the needle is in proper position, the end of the needle will move in a cephalad direction on inspiration and in a caudal direction on expiration.

g. Determine the depth of the kidney by measuring the distance from the needle tip to where it exits the skin.

h. Remove the locating needle and advance the Silverman or Tru-cut needle into the kidney at the same angle and depth as the locating needle using the techniques described in sections II.A or II.B.

7. Complications and Management:

a. Bleeding and hematomas
  • Apply firm direct pressure to puncture sites immediately following aspiration.
  • Correct coagulation abnormalities.

b. Infection
  • Antibiotics as appropriate
  • Incision and drainage as necessary
  • Operative drainage as necessary

c. Pneumothorax
  • More likely in thin patients and deep lesions
  • If tension pneumothorax suspected, decompression with 16 gauge IV into second intercostal space and then tube thoracostomy (see Chapter 3).
  • If 10–20% pneumothorax, observation and serial chest X-rays.
  • If >20% pneumothorax, tube thoracostomy per Chapter 3.

APPENDIX A
LIFE SUPPORT PROTOCOLS

Author: Stephen A. Barnes, M.D.

ADVANCED CARDIAC LIFE SUPPORT (ACLS)[1,2]

Cardiac arrest, and its associated arrhythmias, occurs most commonly outside of the hospital. Nevertheless, the frequency of sudden cardiac death and "malignant" arrhythmias in hospitalized patients is sufficiently high to warrant a basic understanding of cardiopulmonary resuscitation techniques for all house staff. Early intervention is the cornerstone to successful treatment of cardiopulmonary arrest, as early defibrillation or pharmacologic therapy often prevents the initiating arrhythmia from decaying into preterminal states such as ventricular fibrillation or asystole. In descending order of frequency, the primary mechanisms of cardiopulmonary arrest in hospitalized patients are ventricular tachycardia, ventricular fibrillation, and bradycardia. Secondary mechanisms of cardiopulmonary arrest occur when the patient is successfully converted out of ventricular fibrillation and include ventricular tachycardia, bradyarrhythmias such as electromechanical dissociation (EMD) and asystole, and supraventricular arrhythmias.

Common to the treatment of all arrhythmias are an initial assessment and management of the *A, B, C's* (airway, breathing, and circulation), intravenous access, and endotracheal intubation for unstable patients. When possible, intravenous access should be established via a central line placed in the supradiaphragmatic venous system, although large bore antecubital intravenous lines are also acceptable. When intravenous access is impossible or delayed, the following medications can be administered through the endotracheal tube: *naloxone* (if narcotic overdose is suspected), *atropine*, *Valium* (if seizures coincide with the arrest), *epinephrine*, and *lidocaine* (remember mneumonically as "NAVEL"). New algorithms for managing cardiopulmonary arrest were established in 1992. The main modifications to previous protocols were (1) administration of magnesium sulfate to selected patients, (2) use of high dose epinephrine (2.0–2.5 mg) if an initial standard dose fails, or if it is administered via an endotracheal tube, and (3) the limitation of sodium bicarbonate to specific instances. Most authors agree that CPR should be terminated if no rhythm is established after 30 minutes. This time limit should be extended for children, hypothermic and drowning victims, and patients who suffer from recurrent ventricular fibrillation episodes during resuscitation.

The algorithms that follow assume that preliminary efforts have been made to evaluate the patient (i.e., vital signs, history of event) and stabilize him or her (supplemental oxygen, central intravenous access). Throughout the protocols, vital signs should be continually reevaluated, and chest compressions with assisted ventilation instituted whenever cardiopulmonary collapse remains evident.

ADVANCED TRAUMA LIFE SUPPORT (ATLS)[3]

Trauma remains the leading cause of death for individuals of age 1–44 years and ranks third in causing mortality in all age groups. Annually, 3.6 million individuals are hospitalized for injuries directly related to trauma, and the cost in both economic terms and human suffering is enormous. Since the 1970s, a large-scale effort has been made to develop a comprehensive system for the evaluation and treatment of traumatic injuries, the current result of which is found in the American College of Surgeons' Advanced Trauma Life Support. The goals of ATLS are to provide a logical foundation for assessing trauma patients rapidly and accurately, resuscitating and stabilizing patients on a priority basis, and assuring optimum care at each step of the evaluation process.

Proper treatment of trauma patients begins with adequate preparation of the trauma bay and the medical personnel. This includes proper intubation and intravenous access equipment, warm intravenous crystalloid solutions, and institution of universal precautions with waterproof gowns, gloves, masks, and eye shields. Upon arrival in the trauma bay, the evaluation of a patient proceeds systematically to include:

(1) *A primary survey of the A, B, C, D, E's.* Airway, Breathing, Circulation, Disability, and Exposure are evaluated in that order and pathology is treated as soon as it is identified;

(2) *resuscitation* is undertaken with appropriate ventilatory and circulatory support;

(3) *a secondary survey*, consisting of a head-to-toe examination of the patient, follows the initial stabilization efforts;

(4) *monitoring and reevaluation* of the primary and secondary surveys; and

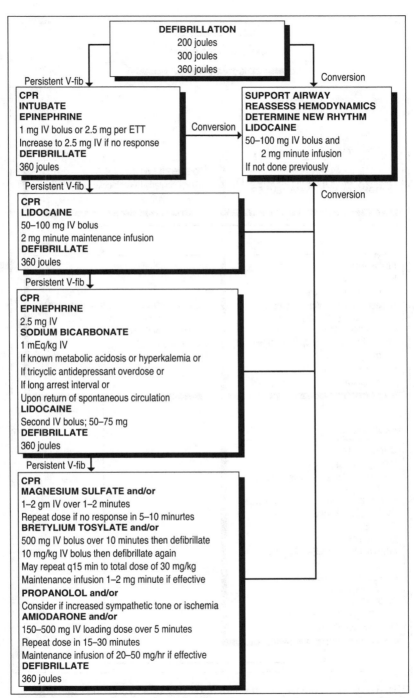

FIGURE 1. Algorithm for treatment of adult ventricular fibrillation. Modified from Grauer K, Cavallaro D. An approach to the key algorithms for cardio-pulmonary resuscitation. In: Welmer RA, Scardiglia J, eds. ACLS Certification Preparation. St. Louis: Mosby Lifeline, 1993:3–38.

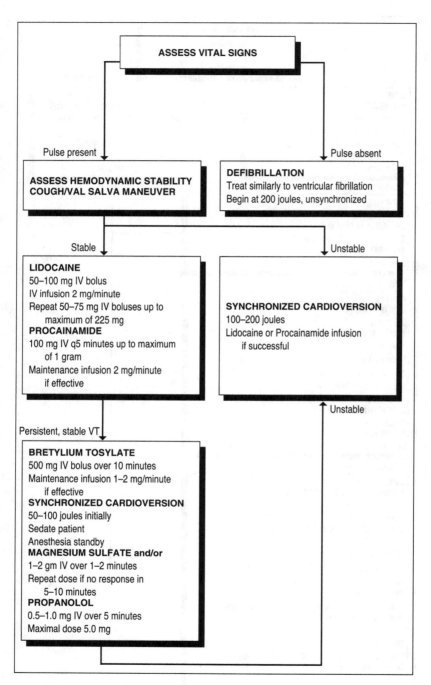

FIGURE 2. Algorithm for treatment of adult sustained ventricular tachycardia. Modified from Grauer K, Cavallaro D. An approach to the key algorithms for cardiopulmonary resuscitation. In: Welmer RA, Scardiglia J, eds. ACLS Certification Preparation. St. Louis: Mosby Lifeline, 1993:3–38.

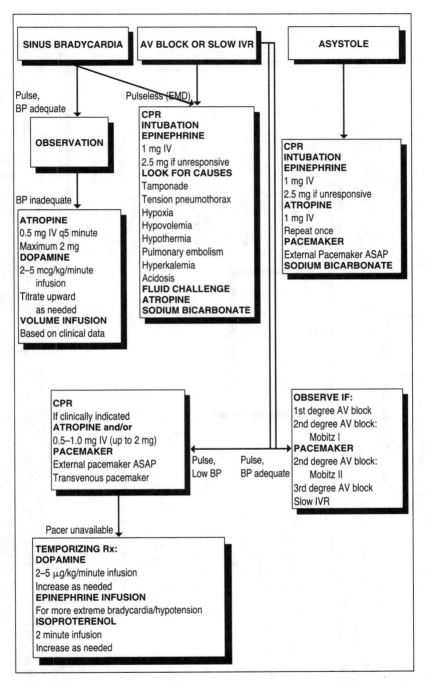

FIGURE 3. Algorithm for treatment of adult bradycardia, EMD, and asystole. Modifed from Grauer K, Cavallaro D. An approach to the key algorithms for cardiopulmonary resuscitation. In: Welmer RA, Scardiglia J, eds. ACLS Certification Preparation. St. Louis: Mosby Lifeline, 1993:3–38.

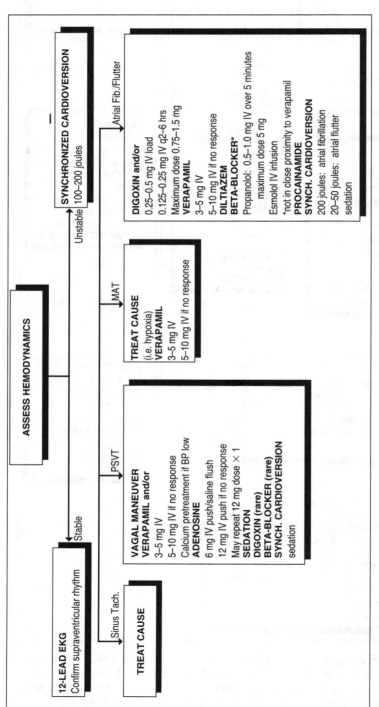

FIGURE 4. Algorithm for treatment of adult supraventricular tachyarrhythmias. Modifed from Grauer K, Cavallaro D. An approach to the key algorithms for cardiopulmonary resuscitation. In: Welmer RA, Scardiglia J, eds. ACLS Certification Preparation. St. Louis: Mosby Lifeline, 1993:3–38. *Legend: PSVT,* paroxysmal supraventricular tachycardia; *MAT,* multifocal atrial tachycardia.

(5) *definitive care* is delivered to any injured organ systems (i.e., operation, casting).

I. PRIMARY SURVEY

A. AIRWAY:
The patient's airway is evaluated and protected if necessary, while concomitantly controlling movement of the cervical spine. In general, if the patient is capable of unstrained speech, his airway is patent. All patients receive supplemental oxygen by mask upon arrival.

1. Clear the Airway:

Finger sweep, then chin lift or jaw thrust.

2. Protect the Airway:

Intubation is indicated when any of the following occur:
a. Apnea
b. Risk of aspiration
c. Impending or actual airway compromise (inhalation injuries, maxillofacial trauma)
d. Closed head injuries (allows hyperventilation to decrease intracranial pressure [ICP])
e. Failure to oxygenate despite supplemental O_2
f. Dislodging of endotracheal tube placed in the field (common)

3. Oropharyngeal Intubation:

Obtunded patient, no obvious C-spine abnormality. Allows larger caliber tube to be placed.

4. Nasopharyngeal Intubation:

Alert, cooperative patient, or when C-spine appears fractured

5. Surgical Airway:

Indicated when there is an inability to intubate the patient
a. Jet ventilation: with small caliber catheter
b. Cricothyroidotomy (standard emergency surgical airway)

6. Cervical Spine Control:

Fundamental at all times during airway management

a. If immobilization devices are unavailable, manual in-line traction is necessary.

b. The cervical spine should be considered unstable (pending radiological investigation) if
   - Physical exam reveals bony abnormalities or the patient complains of spinal tenderness.
   - The patient has experienced multisystem trauma, a blunt injury above the clavicle, or an altered level of consciousness from the trauma or from drug/alcohol intake.
   - Maxillofacial trauma is present.

c. Radiologic evaluation: at least *three views* of the C-spine (lateral, AP, and odontoid)

7. Associated Injuries of the Upper Airway:

Include tracheal and laryngeal disruptions

B. BREATHING AND VENTILATION:

Evaluation of the patient's lungs, chest wall, and diaphragm

1. Tension Pneumothorax:

Needle decompression followed by tube thoracostomy

2. Flail Chest:

Contiguous rib fractures. Danger is associated with underlying pulmonary contusion,

3. Massive Hemothorax:

Control by thoracostomy and/or thoracotomy

4. Open Pneumothorax:

Collapse of involved lung. Control with tube thoracostomy.

5. Other:

Rib fractures, simple pneumothorax, isolated pulmonary contusion

6. Serial Assessments:

Monitor ventilatory rate, ABGs, pulse oximetry.

C. CIRCULATION:

Assessment of patient's central and peripheral blood flow

1. Shock:

Hemorrhagic (most common), cardiogenic (tamponade, my-ocardial trauma), neurogenic (spinal cord injury), septic (rare in acute trauma). Also associated with tension pneumothorax due to decreased venous return to the heart.

2. Hemorrhagic Shock Classification:

a. Class I: <15% blood volume loss. Few if any symptoms
b. Class II: 15–30% blood volume loss. May have tachycardia, anxiety. Responds to intravenous fluids. Note: Tachycardia may be masked if the patient is taking beta-blockers.
c. Class III: 30–40% blood volume loss. Tachycardia, pallor, altered level of consciousness, BP changes
d. Class IV: >40% blood volume loss. Profound cardiovascular collapse, level of consciousness changes

3. Interventions:

a. Two large-caliber (16 gauge or larger) peripheral IVs. May also use central line cordis. Preferred sites are above diaphragm (i.e., antecubital, internal jugular, subclavian veins).
b. Send patient's blood for type and cross, chemistries, and B-hCG (in females).
c. Ringer's lactate infusion (bolus, repeated) "3:1 rule": crystalloid needed = 3 × blood loss
d. Type-specific blood or O negative blood for type III and type IV hemorrhagic shock
e. Control bleeding with direct pressure if possible. Sites of "hidden hemorrhages":
   • Intra-abdominal
   • Intra-thoracic
   • Femur and pelvic fractures
f. Cardiovascular monitoring for arrhythmias and blood pressure, pulse changes
g. Warm fluids and blankets to prevent hypothermia

D. DISABILITY:
Brief neurological assessment.

1. AVPU Evaluation

Based on patient's best response capabilities:
Alert and interactive
Vocal stimuli elicit a response
Painful stimuli are necessary to evoke a response
Unresponsive

Provides only cursory neurological information. A more detailed
assessment utilizing the Glasgow Coma Scale (GCS) is performed
during the secondary survey.

2. Common Etiologies of Neurological Deficits Related to Trauma

a. Closed head injury
b. Hypoxia
c. Shock
d. Alcohol or drug ingestion: category of exclusion (a, b, and c
   must be ruled out).

E. EXPOSURE:
Refers to three evaluations and interventions: exposure of the
patient by undressing, exposure by monitoring and X-rays, and
both historical and incident exposure.

1. Undress the Patient:

a. Remove all clothing, jewelry, etc.
b. Place urinary catheter (Foley). Urine output allows estimate
   of patient's volume status. Contraindications: urethral damage especially in male patients, due to longer urethra
   • Blood at penile meatus
   • Blood/ecchymosis of scrotum
   • High-riding prostate on rectal exam
c. Place nasogastric tube: decompresses stomach and may prevent emesis and aspiration. Contraindications: maxillofacial
   trauma. Cribriform plate fracture may allow nasogastric
   tube to pass into brain. If facial fractures are suspected, use
   an orogastric tube.

2. Monitor and X-Ray the Patient:

a. Ventilation and oxygenation by respiratory rate, ABG, pulse
   oximetry

    b. Cardiovascular status by serial pulse and blood pressured checks. ECG monitor.

    c. X-rays should be obtained once the patient is stabilized. Do not delay evaluation and resuscitation while waiting for X-rays.
- Blunt trauma: C-spine, AP chest, and AP pelvis x-rays are mandatory.
- Penetrating trauma: AP chest and X-rays of trauma site, if applicable.
- After resuscitation is complete, comprehensive X-ray series such as lumbosacral spine and extremity films can be obtained. CT scanning is also performed at this point.

3. Obtain Patient and Incident History:

    a. An "AMPLE" history of the patient includes:
- *Allergies*
- *Medications*
- *Past* medical/surgical history
- *Last* meal
- *Exposures* (past and present) such as tetanus immunization, alcohol/drugs, etc.

    b. The *incident* history should be obtained from the patient and paramedics, if possible.
- Blunt trauma: estimated speed of vehicle, vector, damage, steering wheel deformity, status of windshield, fate of other occupants and crash victims.
- Penetrating trauma: bullet caliber, distance from shooter, number of shots heard
- Burns: associated smoke inhalation, explosion, falling objects, chemicals or toxins
- Cold or heat exposure

II. SECONDARY SURVEY

The secondary survey consists of a head-to-toe examination of the patient and is undertaken once resuscitation efforts are underway and preliminary X-rays have been evaluated.

A. HEAD:

Check for external signs of head injury, scalp lacerations

B. MAXILLOFACIAL:
Assess for stability, fractures, airway patency

C. CERVICAL SPINE:
If the cervical spine films reveal no fracture or dislocation, and the patient is alert and non-intoxicated, the collar can be removed. *Note:* if palpation or range-of-motion reveals tenderness, replace the collar and obtain full radiologic evaluation of the cervical spine. Often this requires CT scanning.

D. NECK:
Evaluate for carotid or tracheolaryngeal trauma.

E. CHEST:
Palpate all ribs for tenderness, assess symmetrical expansion, auscultate all lung fields and heart sounds (decreased in tamponade).

F. ABDOMEN:
Auscultate and palpate four quadrants, assess penetrating injuries.

1. Absolute Indications for Celiotomy:
a. Gunshot wounds to the abdomen
b. Stab wounds that have penetrated the abdominal fascia
c. Expanding abdomen, with or without increase in abdominal pain or fall in blood pressure

2. Further Workup
Consists of CT scan or peritoneal lavage, and is indicated for patients with:
a. Unexplained fall in blood pressure
b. Neurological injury, which may prevent the patient from feeling pain in the abdomen
c. Pelvic or lower rib fractures, which are often associated with trauma to abdominal organs
d. Alcohol or drug use, which dulls the patient's response to pain
e. Equivocal findings on abdominal examination

3. Peritoneal lavage

a. Allows quick evaluation in trauma bay, with full resuscitation equipment nearby
b. Sensitivity approaches 98% (may miss retroperitoneal injuries)
c. Positive if gross blood, >100,000 RBC/hpf, or enteric contents are returned
d. Contraindications:
  - Absolute: obvious need for celiotomy
  - Relative: previous abdominal operations, obesity, cirrhosis, coagulopathy

4. CT scan

a. More fully evaluates retroperitoneal structures and potential pelvic fractures
b. Overall less sensitive but more specific than peritoneal lavage for intraperitoneal injuries
c. Requires transport to scanner, away from full resuscitation equipment
d. Despite potential disadvantages, in centers equipped for rapid CT evaluation, this method of abdominal evaluation may be the procedure of choice.

G. PERINEUM:

Observe for hematoma, perform pelvic exam in females and rectal exam in all patients.

H. MUSCULOSKELETAL:

Pelvic rocking may elicit pain in patients with fractures; evaluate all extremities. Missed extremity fractures are quite common, especially if the patient has multi-system trauma. Occasionally, occult pelvic fractures will not be discovered until the patient feels pain when attempting to walk.

I. NEUROLOGICAL:

Evaluate pupils, cranial nerves, sensation/motor activity in extremities, rectal tone

1. Glasgow Coma Scale (GCS)

a. Assessment of eye opening (1–4)
b. Assessment of verbal response (1–5)

    c. Assessment of motor response (1–6)
    d. Perfect score is 15.
    e. Potential for severe CNS injury is high if GCS <9, moderate if between 9–12

2. CT Scan

Procedure of choice if CNS injury, epidural or subdural hematoma is suspected

3. Paralysis or Paresis

Warrants immediate immobilization and workup for spinal cord trauma

REFERENCES

1. Grauer K, Cavallaro D. An approach to the key algorithms for cardiopulmonary resuscitation. In: Welmer RA, Scardiglia J, eds. ACLS Certification Preparation. St. Louis: Mosby Lifeline, 1993:3–38.
2. American Heart Association, Emergency Cardiac Care Committee and Subcommittees. Guidelines for cardiopulmonary resuscitation and emergency cardiac care. JAMA 1992;268:2171–2295.
3. Alexander R, Proctor H. Advanced trauma life support course for physicians. Chicago: American College of Surgeons Committee on Trauma, 1993:9–396.

APPENDIX B
IV SEDATION

Author: Jay H. Epstein, M.D.

Compassion dictates that patients be provided with anesthesia (analgesia + amnesia) for painful or uncomfortable procedures. Outside of the operating room or ICU, greater caution must be exercised when patients are sedated without expert airway backup nearby, due to the danger of respiratory depression.

A. SYSTEMIC ANALGESICS

1. Morphine:

Reliable opioid that is carefully titrated to clinical effect while the patient is closely monitored for respiratory depression.

    a. Dose: IV/IM: 1–2 mg titrated every 8 minutes
    b. Onset: IV: 30 seconds; IM: 2–5 minutes
    c. Peaks: IV: Analgesia in 3–4 minutes, respiratory depression in 15 minutes; IM: 45 minutes
    d. Duration: IV/IM: 2–7 hours
    e. Side Effects: Cardiovascular and respiratory depression, bronchospasm, urinary retention, constipation, pruritus
    f. Comments: Dose cautiously in the elderly or hypovolemic patient. Hypotensive/respiratory depression synergistic with other CNS acting drugs (benzodiazepines, for example). Partial reversal of sedative effect by naloxone.

2. Fentanyl (sublimaze):

An alternative for patients with a true morphine allergy, Fentanyl is also more useful than morphine in COPD patients due to its propensity to cause less histamine release.

    a. Dose: 25–50 μg IV titrated every six minutes
    b. Onset: 30 seconds
    c. Peaks: IV Analgesic peak in 2–3 minutes, respiratory depression in 10 minutes

d. Duration: 30–60 minutes

e. Side Effects/Comments: As above for morphine.

3. Ketorolac (Toradol):

The first IV nonsteroidal anti-inflammatory agent, ketorolac is a good choice (in eligible patients) on its own or as an adjunct with narcotics. Ketorolac 30 mg is equal analgesic to morphine 10 mg, and has no respiratory depression properties.

a. Dose: IV: 60 mg load, then 30 mg IV every 6 hours, for total of 72 hours only; reduce dose 50% in patients >65 years old.

b. Onset: 10 minutes

c. Peaks: 45 minutes

d. Duration: 2–6 hours

e. Side Effects: Inhibits platelet function and decreases renal perfusion

f. Comments: Contraindicated in patients with renal insufficiency (Cr >1.5 mg/dl); cautious use in patients older than 65.

B. SEDATION/AMNESTIC AGENTS

1. Midazolam (Versed):

Rapid acting benzodiazepine that is titrated to clinical effect.

a. Dose: IV: 0.5–1.0 mg titrated every 4–5 minutes

b. Onset: 1 minute

c. Peaks: 10 minutes

d. Duration: 1–2 hours

e. Side Effects: Cardiovascular and respiratory depression possible; paradoxical disinhibition may occur in elderly patients

f. Comments: Dose cautiously in the elderly or hypovolemic patient; dangerously synergistic with other CNS acting drugs (opioids, for example); partial reversal of effect with flumazenil.

2. Diazepam (Valium):

Longer acting, but slightly more difficult to titrate to effect than midazolam.

a. Dose: IV: 0.5–2 mg increments, titrated every 5–6 minutes

b. Onset: 3–5 minutes

c. Peaks: 5–10 minutes

d. Duration: 2–3 hours

e. Side Effects/Comments: As above for midazolam; painful upon injection, give only IV, in divided doses.

3. Haloperidol (Haldol):

A butyrophenone antipsychotic with little cardiorespiratory depression, haloperidol is an excellent sedative for the acutely ill patient.
   a. Dose: IV: 0.5–1.0 mg, titrating in 1–4 mg every 8 minutes
   b. Onset: 2–3 minutes
   c. Peaks: 5–15 minutes
   d. Duration: 45–180 minutes
   e. Side Effects: Tardive dyskinesia (rare), neuroleptic malignant syndrome (rare)

C. REVERSAL AGENTS

1. Flumazenil (Mazicon):

Works as a benzodiazepine antagonist
   a. Dose: IV: 0.2 mg every minute up to 1.0 mg; maximum of 3 mg in one hour
   b. Onset: 1–2 minutes
   c. Peaks: 5–10 minutes
   d. Duration: 45–90 minutes
   e. Side Effects: Excessive catecholamine state secondary to reversal of sedation; seizures in predisposed patients (those with seizure or alcohol/sedative abuse histories)
   f. Comments: Resedation may occur secondary to residual benzodiazepine; IV drip of 30–60 μg/min may be required for several hours until the drug is fully metabolized.

2. Naloxone (Narcan): An antagonist at the opioid receptor

   a. Dose: IV: 20–40 μg every 5 minutes until reversal of narcotization achieved
   b. Onset: 1–5 minutes
   c. Peaks: 7 minutes
   d. Duration: 30–60 minutes
   e. Side Effects: Excessive catecholamine state secondary to reversal of analgesia and return of pain
   f. Comments: Resedation may occur secondary to residual narcotization; IV drip of 20–80 μg/hr may be required until opioid fully metabolized.

APPENDIX C
INFORMED CONSENT

Author: C. Max Schmidt, M.D., M.B.A.

Informed consent is a concept that can be broken down into two parts: informing and consenting. To be informed means to comprehend the course of action and its consequences. This comprehension almost invariably comes from a physician's dialogue with the patient. Consent means to express a willingness to proceed or not proceed with a specific course of action. In addition, informed consent is a contextual concept and is only valid in a specific context. Therefore, informed consent is an expression of one's understanding and willingness to proceed or not to proceed with certain actions in a specific context. Conversely, if the patient is unwilling, does not understand, or the specific context is altered, informed consent is invalid. It is not in the patient's best interest to proceed and the physician can be liable for battery and/or negligence for proceeding under these circumstances.

Application of the working definition of informed consent to the context of bedside procedures gives a more practical definition for the physician. Informed consent is written, verbal, and/or implied testimony that a given individual understands and wills the procedure planned as well as possible modifications to the planned procedure, its indications, predictable outcomes (i.e., the effectiveness of the procedure and operator and predictable consequences of the procedure whether adverse or beneficial), possible complications (severity and frequency of occurrence), and alternative therapies and their respective costs/benefits in the patient's specific context.

Having established the definitional constraints of informed consent, several necessary conditions remain to ensure that informed consent is achieved. These conditions are a competent physician and patient, critical information delivery, and an elective setting.

A competent physician is one who understands the diagnosis, the prognosis, and the nature, purpose, outcomes, risks, benefits, and alternatives of the procedure and is able to confer these in layman terms without substantially altering their meaning or significance to the patient. If the physician understands the procedure and its actual and potential consequences and has ready access to specific details (not necessarily committed to memory) then he or she may feel comfortable serving as the responsible informant for the patient. In the past, physician competence for this process has been determined solely by introspection, peer review, and professional standards. Legal and economic sanctions, however, have encouraged third parties to make it their business to ensure quality controls.

Another requirement of informed consent is the delivery of critical information. At the minimum the law's standard of disclosure should be followed. The law's standard used to be based upon the standard of care as established by the medical profession. It is now based upon the informational needs of an average, reasonable person (Canterbury v. Spence, 464 F.2d 772, 780: D.C. Cir. 1972). An immediate consideration then is that the information be delivered in simple, nontechnical terms. The physician informant must be careful, however, that in so doing he does not alter the meaning and significance of the information.

The information delivered should include an explanation of the diagnosis and the indications, nature, and purpose of the procedure. Explanation of diagnosis and indications for the procedure should include differentiation between true, working, differential, and no diagnoses and how the discovery of alternative diagnoses affect therapy and outcome. Explanation of the nature and purpose of treatment should be succinct and not dwell on specific technical details of the case. Such details are important for the surgeon to understand but the patient should not be involved in this decision-making except where patient preference may modify techniques that directly affect outcomes. An illustration is often a helpful instructional tool and also is good evidence in the permanent medical record that an intelligent and detailed discussion took place preoperatively. Consent is limited to those procedures contemplated when consent is given, so prior consent to necessary or possible extensions of the original procedure are recommended. Also, informed consent is limited to specific named practitioners; otherwise, it is considered misrepresentation.

Disclosure of risks and consequences of treatment has been the subject of much litigation in the area of informed consent. Events with a significant probability of occurrence or significant severity (regardless of the probability) should be disclosed. The actual risk probabilities in general (and specific to the proposed operator if significantly different) should be disclosed if known. In today's legalistic environment the physician, when explaining risks, should sway towards full disclosure of risks. Conversely, therapeutic privilege (i.e., the option of nondisclosure of information that may affect an irrational decision on the part of the patient or may theoretically harm the patient's psychological well being) should not be exercised unless overwhelming evidence from multiple credible sources supports this method of reserved disclosure.

The probability of success of the procedure must be discussed with the patient. This includes the general probability (as well as the specific operator's probability if significantly different) of successful completion of the procedure, the probability that this particular procedure will achieve the desired and stated outcomes, and the probability of necessary future surgery as a result of the proposed procedure. Treatment alternatives deemed feasible by the medical community should be disclosed with their respective nature, purpose, outcomes, risks, benefits, and prognosis. Finally, the patient's prognosis without the proposed treatment should be conferred.

Another requirement of informed consent is a competent patient of legal age. If there is any question about a patient's competence or ability to understand the procedure and its ramifications, the procedure should be postponed until the physician and others involved make a full evaluation of the patient's mental status. The evaluation should help determine the most appropriate action whether it is legally approved substitute consent, postponement of procedure until patient recovers competent status, or cancellation of the procedure. Documenting patient competency is sometimes a tedious process and, therefore, should not be delayed. Legally approved substitute consent is usually in the order of spouse, parent, child (if legal age), sibling, then other relatives. If the patient has no family member to legally substitute consent, then the incompetent patient becomes the legal responsibility of the state and a guardian is appointed to make these decisions on the patient's behalf. If there is ever a question of who can or cannot be a legally approved substitute, especially in light of a certain family's social situations, acquire legal consultation. And, finally, if any decision by a legally approved substitute seems inappropriate and perhaps detrimental to the patient's care, then address the matter with the legal office. There are times when such a decision can be overridden.

A final requirement is an elective setting. Thorough and effective delivery of information and time for a patient to absorb its significance and import is not practical or possible in an emergent setting. Under such circumstances the patient must trust and the physician must act. Although a medical emergency may obviate the need for consent, it is still advisable, however, to inform patient and family expediently of the patient's critical condition and current therapeutic plans. In these circumstances, although not necessary, an "administrative consent" may be obtained through the legal counsel or administrator on-call for the hospital. This philosophy is applicable to the elective setting as well, for it is important to not hurry or rush through the process of consent. For example, obtaining consent from a patient in the preoperative holding area or with other fairly inflexible time constraints is generally a poor practice.

The consent form in and of itself is not a legal document and serves more or less as a checklist or guide for physician patient interaction. JCAH (Joint Commission for Accreditation of Hospitals), however, requires informed consent as part of the patient's medical record. The process of informed consent obviously has huge legal implications and therefore must be taken very seriously. Obtaining informed consent is necessary but not sufficient to free one from liability. Any bedside procedure must have the consent of the patient. The intentional touching of another person without express consent of the individual is "battery." Consent for certain procedures such as blood draws or peripheral IV starts in an awake and interactive patient are verbal and/or implied consents. More extensive procedures should, however, have a written consent form and a note in the chart documenting the discussion that took place prior to the procedure or treatment. Written consent provides the most direct, effective proof of consent. If one forgets to have a patient sign a consent document, the most important thing to do is write a note in the chart documenting your discussion with the patient and their willingness to proceed. Court cases where this issue has come up suggest that in an awake and interactive patient, consent is implied regardless of whether they signed a hospital form (i.e., the patient at any time could have refused the treatment and chose not to); therefore, consent is implied from the circumstances. Most importantly, keep patients and families informed for the purpose of providing the best care to them possible.

ADEQUATE SUPERVISION

There are no strictly adhered to standards for adequate supervision of bedside procedures at any hospitals with residency programs. One reason for this may be that there is little data to support one method over another in terms of patient outcomes. In general senior house staff as well as attending staff should be responsible for ensuring that junior house staff and medical students are well supervised and feel comfortable performing bedside procedures. Furthermore, supervision of bedside procedures should not be exclusive to the actual technical task of performing the procedure. Supervision should also extend to the preoperative assessment, proper consent of the patient, the procedure itself, and diagnostic and therapeutic management of postoperative complications. The ultimate responsibility of ensuring adequate supervision rests on the individual performing the procedure. Each physician must determine from their experience and skill level their degree of comfort with the procedure and seek help or supervision accordingly.

Supervision of physicians in training performing bedside procedures should begin with the supervision of their preoperative assessments. Patient's clinical situations are multiple and diverse in a complex medical, ethical, and legal environment. No procedure should be performed on a patient without proper preoperative assessment. Nor should a procedure be performed by a physician who does not understand the preoperative assessment.

Supervision of preoperative assessments helps physicians in training to begin to understand the proper indications and contraindications to procedures and how they vary with individual patients. Based upon the patient's history, physical and pertinent laboratory and radiographic data, the physician must determine whether the procedure is indicated and whether the risk/benefit profile is acceptable. Even if the patient's medical condition indicates, the physician must consider other factors which optimize one's ability to perform a safe and effective procedure (e.g., time constraints, time of day, equipment limitations, patient cooperation, nursing staff resources, and senior house officer or attending availability). The margin for error escalates when conditions are not optimal. In cases where the physician does not believe the procedure is indicated or believes that it is contraindicated in light of the risk/benefit profile, he or she should not perform the procedure. The patient's case should be reviewed by the primary care providers and the patient to come to an optimal solution. Supervision of physicians obtaining informed consent is the next important step. Experience will ultimately provide the best education for the physician on how to effectively communicate with different patients and their families.

After preoperative assessment and informed consent are accomplished, the physician's technical abilities should be supervised. "See one, do one, teach one" has no place here. Everyone's abilities differ and each procedure require different levels of skill and experience. It is therefore difficult to set down firm guidelines. As an example, the guidelines for subclavian vein central line placement may be to observe five, perform 20 in the elective setting under strict supervision, 20 with supervision readily available if needed, then, finally, self-supervised. The physician in training should look objectively at the type and frequency of complications of procedures where he or she was the principal operator and modify technique accordingly. Even the most experienced operators occasionally struggle with seemingly routine procedures. Don't be persistent or stubborn at the expense of patient comfort and safety. Finally, the physician in training must be supervised until competent at the post-operative management of complications of bedside procedures. This means the ability to diagnose, expedite, and perform appropriate therapy.

In summary, optimal supervision of bedside procedures should not be exclusive to the technical task itself but include the preoperative assessment, consent of the patient, the technical aspects of the procedure itself, and diagnostic and therapeutic management of postoperative complications. The ultimate responsibility of ensuring adequate supervision rests on the individual performing the procedure. Each physician must be honest with himself or herself and determine from experience and skill level the degree of comfort with the procedure and seek help or supervision accordingly.

INDEX